Helping language development

A developmental programme for
children with early language handicaps

Helping language development

A developmental programme for children with early language handicaps

Jean Cooper

Molly Moodley

Joan Reynell

Edward Arnold

First published 1978 by
Edward Arnold (Publishers) Ltd.
25 Hill Street, London W1X 8LL

Cooper, Jean
  Helping language development.
  1. Children — language 2. Speech therapy
  3. Communicative disorders in children
  I. Title   II. Moodley, Molly
  III. Reynell, Joan
  371. 9'14   LB1139.L3

ISBN boards: 0 7131 6101 9
        paper: 0 7131 6102 7

Text set in 11 pt Photon Times, printed by photolithography, and bound in Great Britain at The Pitman Press, Bath

Contents

Preface

The procedures described here were developed at The Wolfson Centre, Institute of Child Health, in London, in an attempt to find effective means of helping the children who were referred to this centre with early language handicaps. The project has now reached the stage at which the procedures can be recommended to other people who are professionally concerned with helping such children. The final follow-up studies are not yet complete, and more detailed reports of the research project await further publications. In the meantime, this handbook is intended as a guide to anyone who is interested in using this approach. It is written mainly for speech therapists, teachers, medical practitioners, and psychologists, who are the people most likely to be directing this type of work. Other people concerned with language-handicapped children may be interested, but a certain amount of professional understanding is advisable, and has been assumed in writing the book.

Acknowledgements

This research was supported by a generous grant from the Department of Education and Science.

Very special thanks are due to Sheila Donaldson, speech therapist, who carried out much of the 'parent' programme, and the Heather Soar, nursery assistant, who helped with the language class.

We are also grateful to Professor Holt and the staff of The Wolfson Centre, Institute of Child Health, where the project was based.

1977   Jean Cooper
                                                       Molly Moodley
                                                       Joan Reynell

Chapter 1   Introduction

'Don't worry, he'll grow out of it', 'it will be all right when he gets to school', 'speech therapists can't do anything until he is four years old'. These maxims, common a generation ago, are now rarely encountered in relation to early language handicaps. It has become increasingly recognized that early help is feasible, effective and important. This recognition has led to a number of different programmes designed to provide this early help. These are discussed on pp. 14–16. This volume presents a developmental approach to helping children, an approach which has now had extensive trials and has proved effective in accelerating language development in the great majority of children presenting with early language difficulties.

In the past, most of the emphasis in assessing and helping language development has been on the ability to speak. A failure to develop speech is the most obvious manifestation of a language difficulty, whereas more extensive and perhaps more important aspects of language involvement may go unrecognized. Parents often claim that 'he understands everything I say', not realizing that they are using massive non-verbal situational clues in their communication with their child, so that difficulties in receptive language go unnoticed. By the time a delay in speaking becomes evident, there may already have been more serious difficulties concerned with delay in the development of an understanding of symbols (or representations) (see chapter 2), and in verbal comprehension, both of which can interfere with intellectual development. Language is itself an intellectual process which extends far beyond the ability to talk, and is basic to the healthy development of many other intellectual processes. The developmental programme described here takes account of this broad view of language, and much of the work is concerned with the basic process of symbolic understanding, leading to the understanding of verbal language, and to the use of language in thinking. Assessment takes account of the very early pre-language developmental stages, so that verbal language may be built upon a sound and developmentally appropriate foundation.

Importance of early intervention

Among the most important reasons for helping children as soon as a specific language problem is recognized are:

(1) Language is an intellectual process, which, in the pre-school years, becomes integrated with other intellectual areas so that the whole process of thinking becomes extended and enhanced. The work of Luria (1961), confirmed by many followers, has shown that at about $3\frac{1}{2}$ years of age language becomes important as a directive function for practical activities. By the use of language children become able to plan and monitor their activities with concrete material, so extending their range of abilities. Later, this use of language is internalized so that it becomes a substitute for the action itself, so introducing 'short cuts' to the solution of practical problems.

Francis-Williams (1970) and others have shown that language plays an important part in concept formation. For example, the use of language helps in classifying objects according to abstractions such as colour, size and use. The understanding of the concept 'big' as an attribute, is helped by labelling the concept with a word or sign.

Furth (1966) and others, working with deaf children, have shown that certain intellectual tasks are facilitated by the use of internalized language.

The evidence is overwhelming, and points to the need for helping children to develop enough language to serve these intellectual needs during the years before school starts.

(2) The important years for language development are between $1\frac{1}{2}$ and $4\frac{1}{2}$. There is very rapid language development during these three years. In fact by $4\frac{1}{2}$ years most children have fully established language which can be internalized as a thinking process. It is easier to help language during these three years of development than to try to make up the ground after the age of five years, when other intellectual processes have already outstripped the deviant language and the whole has become skewed. Language should be helped during development, at the normal developmental stage.

(3) The need for easy communication is recognized as basic to healthy social and emotional development. Any interference with this is likely to have far reaching effects. This is, of course, another reason for early intervention, as soon as communication problems are recognized. Good communication between the child and his family forms the basis for healthy relationships. If a difficulty in understanding verbal communication goes unrecognized, this can lead to behaviour difficulties such as apparently 'obstinate' or negative responses, or a failure to conform, which can disturb the whole family equilibrium. This can occur long before the child is expected to talk, so is often not recognized as due to a communication failure. Later, when the child wants to make himself un-

derstood, frustration occurs if he cannot communicate his needs. This can lead to tantrums and perhaps destructive and antisocial behaviour. If the communication difficulties persist into school age, there are additional problems arising from a failure of communication with peers and teachers, and difficulties with the verbal aspects of school learning. Communication within the family, and later with peers and teachers, is as essential to healthy social and emotional development as it is to academic achievement. If language difficulties can be recognized and helped at an early stage, many of these difficulties may be prevented.

Types of language handicap

In deciding on the type of provision needed for children with early language handicaps, it has been helpful to use the following three categories, while recognizing that there may be a considerable overlap between them. Children in the first category, environmental delay, can probably be helped equally well by ordinary nursery-school methods, or in a good day nursery, but children in the second and third categories need special help and do well with the developmental programme.

(1) *Environmental language delay:* This is an environmentally caused language delay in otherwise normal children, usually resulting from inadequate early language experience (some sort of 'deprivation'), or from a non-English speaking home (Randall, Reynell and Curwen 1974). This type of delay is not often severe, and it usually resolves spontaneously with appropriate learning opportunities such as ordinary nursery school may provide. These children have not been included in our work on the developmental programme unless there was evidence that they also had a developmental language handicap. Children from a foreign-speaking home who demonstrate delay in all aspects of language including their native tongue, would be suitable candidates for the programme.

(2) *Developmental language delay:* This is a constitutionally determined developmental handicap. It may be mild or severe, and may or may not be associated with evidence of a more generally handicapping condition. This amounts to a handicap needing special help when receptive and/or expressive language development is not more than two-thirds of the nonverbal intellectual abilities in terms of age level. Although this is a serious and pathological delay, the language, when it appears, follows a fairly consistent developmental pattern, following the normal stages of early language development. The natural history of this type of language delay is for verbal comprehension and expressive language to be approximately equally delayed at first, often with very immature attention control. Verbal comprehension recovers first, then the more central aspects of expressive language (words and sentences), and finally the more mature

coding of sounds in words (intelligibility) (Reynell 1972). Early intonation patterns and the stages of development of speech sounds are usually
normal but delayed in these children (Ward 1973). Children with this
type of language delay need special help in the pre-school years so that
they are not at risk for delay in the intellectual processes which depend
on language.

(3) *Developmental language disorder:* These children also have a severe
and specific language delay, but the pattern of their language is not only
delayed but deviant. There is no clear pattern of recovery, as in (2)
above, but development is uneven and atypical. The handicap may be
very specifically concerned with one aspect of language, for example a
specific type of receptive or expressive difficulty. Verbal comprehension
may or may not be entirely normal. The handicap is sometimes difficult
to overcome completely. Such children often (but not always) have a
clear and demonstrable extension of the handicap to other areas, such as
neurological signs. These children have been included in our studies.
They usually make good early progress but complete recovery is slower
than in (2) above, and they may enter school with a disability still severe
enough to need on-going help.

Categories (2) and (3) may show considerable overlap, and the pattern
may change as the child gets older. A good deal of work still needs to be
done before early language handicaps can be confidently separated in
this way, and it has only been attempted here as a very broad division.
Further work on this aspect is in progress. As far as providing help is
concerned, both groups do well in the developmental language
programme as this is directed towards the more basic stages of language
development, common to all such handicaps.

Review of other programmes

The literature on language disabilities in children is rapidly expanding
and contains many and various descriptions of language programmes
and management approaches. Most of these appear to be concerned
specifically with the verbal communication processes and do not
necessarily extend in any depth to the intellectual processes involved in
language. They are aimed at the development of expressive language, articulation, syntax and spoken vocabulary, and although acknowledging
the importance of verbal comprehension do not emphasize this aspect in
their approach to the remediation of the problem. There are exceptions to
this and some of these are referred to below.

At the risk of over-simplifying the review of this extensive variety of
approaches it seems that they fall into three broad categories, namely
phonetic, syntactic and semantic (Marge (1972) suggested phonetic, syntactic and developmental.)

(1) *Phonetic:* Currently this would seem to be the least popular approach. It is based on an assumption that sounds are the foundations from which words and sentences develop. In such a programme specific training is given in auditory discrimination, exercises of the articulatory mechanism, practice in imitation of speech-sounds in increasingly complex patterns and then practice of these sounds in conversational speech and oral reading.

(2) *Syntactic:* This is perhaps the most popular approach but would seem to be widely interpreted. It can vary from specific practice and drill in the eliciting of basic sentence patterns and expanding these for the child to imitate, to a development of concepts and structured verbalization of experiences and events in the child's daily routine. Notable in this category would be the work of Laura Lee *et al.* (1975), *Interactive language development teaching* and David Crystal *et al.* (1976) *The grammatical analysis of language disability.*

(3) *Semantic:* This approach focuses on enriching the child's experiences and developing his understanding of events from which it is assumed language should develop. It embraces the development of perceptual skills and specific training is given in verbal labelling, vocabulary building and concept development. It is a much less structured approach than either of the preceding two and is again interpreted in a variety of ways.

The setting up and choice of emphasis of these various language programmes often has been influenced by a variety of factors such as the number of personnel available, the training and expertise of that personnel and the physical setting in which the programme is to be carried out. Language intervention programmes take place in the classroom setting, the nursery school, community clinics, hospital clinics, special assessment centres, special schools and the home. This also often influences the design and the manner in which it can be carried out.

It would be wrong to indicate that all language intervention programmes fall into such clearly defined categories of approach. There are many which are more eclectic and are of course modified to the needs of the child's particular language problem whether it be a specific disorder, a constitutional delay or the result of cultural deprivation.

Many of the programmes have originated in the United States and are in fact directed towards the needs of the socially disadvantaged child. A very useful summary and bibliography of such programmes is provided in a book by Walburga Von Raffler-Engel and Robert Hutcheson entitled *Language Intervention Programs in the United States 1960/1974* (1975).

A survey by Courtney Cazden of existing programmes for similar children in England and Wales is given in a book edited by Celia

Lavatelli entitled *Language Training and Early Childhood Education* (1972).

Some programmes designed for the problem of the socially disadvantaged child are adopted for use with children whose language is specifically disordered or constitutionally delayed and would seem to have less value in that context. Examples of this might be the Distar programme and the use of the Peabody Language Kit.

Three further approaches which do not fit into the categories previously mentioned are:

(i) That of Fraser and Blockley (1973): The aim of this programme is said to be 'to develop the child's appreciation of relationship in time and space and his ability to categorize and to form simple concepts.' The authors considered that the language disorder could not be remedied through working in the medium in which the disorder lay (i.e. language) and therefore the programme concentrates on specific training of non-verbal skills largely presented in a non-verbal manner.

(ii) Also in current use is a language programme designed by A. Kirk and W. D. Kirk (1972) which is based upon the model of the Illinois Test of Psycholinguistic Abilities (ITPA).

(iii) The work at the Heston Adrian Research Centre at Manchester University is again different in approach. Here a number of workshops for parents of mentally handicapped children have been organized. The emphasis has been on increasing the parents' and the classroom teachers' ability to utilize everyday learning situations, structuring them to the particular developmental needs of each child. This work contains many of the same principles of the intervention measures described in this handbook. It is however more particularly directed towards general learning difficulties than towards specific language difficulties and is carried out as a workshop during a specified period of time rather than as an on-going clinical and classroom service.

Without attempting to review all the language programmes it can, however, be seen from the foregoing references and comments that these are very varied in design and management and need to be very carefully considered for their appropriateness to the needs of the individual child.

The developmental approach

Aims

The approach to helping language-handicapped children, described in this volume, is not a 'programme' in the usual sense, although this word is used for want of a better one. The word 'programme' suggests too rigid a system, and flexibility is one of the most important features of the developmental approach.

The main features are:

(1) *Developmental/intellectual orientation:* Language is regarded as an intellectual process rather than merely as a means of social interchange. It is understood to cover the whole range of symbolic understanding, and is not confined to a verbal system. Importance is attached to the use of language as a directive-integrative function and to its use in many thought processes. It is important that consideration be given to the integration of language with other intellectual processes at the appropriate developmental stages, so that helping language, in the broadest sense, becomes part of helping intellectual development; and conversely, other intellectual processes may be used to help deviant language. This is discussed further in chapter 3, in relation to the model shown in Figure 2.

(2) *Flexibility:* The system is designed to have extreme flexibility, so that, provided the basic developmental model is understood, the approach may be adapted for parents working with their children at home; for teachers in schools or special units; or for staff in Day Nurseries. It is also individually adaptable in that each child has his own 'programme' tailored to his particular level and pattern of development, which is established at the time of assessment. Field studies (chapter 7) have shown that the approach is effective with children who have wide-ranging intellectual abilities, and with very varied patterns of handicaps.

(3) *Built-in system of recording progress:* The approach is aimed at achieving accelerated language development, while following the normal developmental stages discussed in chapter 3. Progress is recorded stage by stage for each child, by whoever is carrying out the programme, so that a logical sequence is achieved, and progress can be continuously assessed. There is no need to wait for annual reassessment by a psychologist or medical officer, in order to find out what progress has been made. Our studies have shown that these regular records kept by the teacher or speech therapists directing the intervention are better estimates of progress than are the quantitative measures obtained at annual review (see chapter 7). If progress is not seen, it is in any case too late to wait a year. Adaptations must be introduced so that progress is achieved.

Scope and limitations

Studies have shown that the developmental programme can be useful for children with a wide range of handicaps, provided they are intellectually within the pre-school range. Older children, who have a very specific language difficulty, may need a more linguistically structured approach such as some of those mentioned in chapter 1. Deaf children, and children with specific problems in speech production due to poor muscular control, also need a more specific type of help.

It has been possible to help some children with extensive communication problems, children showing autistic features, by this approach, but there have not been extensive trials with these children, and not all of them respond well. In some cases, although the language problem has been helped, behaviour difficulties have persisted, and needed more intensive psychiatric help. It is important to recognize these extended difficulties, and refer the child for further help as appropriate.

Mentally handicapped children usually respond well, and it has been encouraging to see the approach used effectively with some severely subnormal children.

Age range

In general 'the younger the better' is a useful guiding principle. Research has shown that children between 2 and 4 years old make faster progress than those taken on for help at the age of 4+ years. As the programme is developmentally rational, it is appropriate and advisable to introduce such help as soon as a language difficulty can be recognized. This is usually by the age of 2 years, when non-verbal abilities can be seen to be outstripping language. However, the developmental approach is suitable for children of any age, or mental age, from 2 to 5 years.

Who carries out the programme?

The programme needs to be professionally directed by someone, such as a psychologist, speech therapist, medical officer, or specialist teacher, who has a sound understanding of early intellectual and language development. It may be carried out under this direction by people who are in constant contact with the child but who do not necessarily have the basic professional training, such as parents and nursery assistants.

As a specific language delay is often a presenting facet of a more extensive handicapping condition, there is of course a need for the constant supervision of a paediatrician, who forms part of the assessment team (see chapter 4).

In the following pages the intervention programme will be presented as it was carried out in the research project, in the following two ways:

(1) *Language 'clinic' programme:* The teaching was carried out by the parents at home, as part of the process of daily living. One or both parents and child were seen by the speech therapist once in six weeks to reinforce and guide the procedure, and the child was reassessed annually by a psychologist and paediatrician, and sometimes by a medical social worker. This annual reassessment is in addition to the regular progress

records kept by the teachers or speech therapist.

(2) *Language class:* The children attended for two hours a day, five days a week during school term, without their parents. The classes, each of eight children, were under the direction of a qualified teacher assisted by a nursery nurse. Assessments were carried out annually by the professional team as above.

Each child was fully assessed before being taken on. As a result of the assessment an individual programme was established on the basis of the model shown in Figure 2 (p. 27). The task of the person directing the programme was then to consolidate the developmental stage and lead on to the next one while at the same time maintaining a balanced integration between all the processes concerned. This is discussed in more detail in chapter 3.

Creating a language learning environment

'Early education is part of, and integrated with total living. It is not confined to certain hours of the day, or days of the week, but depends on creating a total educational environment so that each child, whatever his handicaps, may be enabled to use each daily living experience to promote and enrich his development. It is the role of those who are professionally concerned with education and development to work with the parents so that this early education may take place in the most appropriate way.' (Reynell 1976a.)

This is the philosophy upon which the developmental programme is based. The more usual half-an-hour a week with a speech therapist is not enough for young children. A week is too long a gap, and a half-hour session too little. Also, it is inappropriate with young children to separate a teaching session from daily living. The developmental language programme depends on adapting the language environment, whether at home or at school, so that it can be an on-going experience all and every day, built in to the daily living routine.

Chapter 2　Language development

As the intervention programme described here is a 'developmental' one, a short description of language development is given in this chapter, to explain the basis of the procedure. Great emphasis is laid on pre-language stages, as an essential foundation for adequate language development. A fuller description of this view of language development and its assessment can be found in Reynell (1976b).

Definitions

'Language' is described in the very broadest sense as an ability to understand and use symbols, particularly verbal symbols, in thinking and as a form of communication. The ability to 'speak' is only one aspect of language, and is less important, developmentally, than the ability to understand language and to use it as a thought process.

A 'symbol' is something which can stand for, or represent something else, such as a picture of a chair, or small toy chair, which can represent the idea or concept of a chair. Developmentally this understanding of symbols enables a child to understand representations with a gradually decreasing perceptual similarity to the object they represent; in other words, symbols which are increasingly 'arbitrary' (Conn 1974). Much of the early 'baby talk' has arisen from the need for a gradual transfer from a perceptually similar symbol to the more abstract word. For example, 'quack-quack' for duck, and 'tick-tock' for clock. A word such as 'chair' has no perceptual similarity to the object chair, and is therefore a highly arbitrary symbol. In order to understand this sort of representation a child must already have achieved a relatively good level of symbolic understanding. If he is taught to 'speak' before this level of understanding is reached, he may use words in the situation in which they were taught, but they will have no meaning for him apart from that particular set of circumstances. This can lead to the repetitive and apparently meaningless type of speech which sometimes occurs with autistic children.

Development of pre-language

(1) *Early concept formation:* There can be no meaningful symbol until

there is something in the child's understanding for the symbol to represent. He must have reached at least the early stages of concept formation before any meaningful language is possible. A concept is an inner awareness of an object, or an idea, which can be carried over when the object is not present. The earliest stages of concept formation begin with the awareness of permanence of objects (Piaget 1953). This is an understanding that an object can continue to exist when it is no longer perceived at the moment. This can usually be demonstrated by the age of nine months by getting the child to search for a desired object which is momentarily hidden from him. When this very basic stage of intellectual development has been reached, the stages leading up to symbolic understanding may follow.

(2) *Situational understanding:* Several months before the development of symbolic understanding, children may demonstrate an understanding of familiar phrases which have been learnt as part of a regularly occurring sequence of events. Such phrases usually have a clear intonation and rhythmic pattern, and are used by a familiar person in a particular situation. The child's response forms part of a well learnt sequence of events, and demonstrates understanding which is limited to this context. A common example is 'give Mummy a kiss', when the child is seated on the mother's knee facing her, and she approaches her face to his. At this stage of understanding the child will respond appropriately to the right person in the right situation, if the phrase is said according to the learnt tonal and rhythmic pattern, but individual words have no meaning. The phrase is only meaningful as part of a familiar sequence of events, and is in no way representational or symbolic.

The same thing happens, developmentally, with expressive pre-language at the stage of jargon. A child will use intonation patterns and rhythms which simulate phrases in certain daily situations. This stage of development usually immediately precedes the first meaningful word.

Older, retarded children may remain at this pre-language stage for a long time, perhaps acquiring quite a large repertoire of phrases which they can use or respond to in the right situations. This can be misleading in terms of their language level unless the stage is understood as pre-language and not representational language.

This pre-language stage is an important way-station to true language, and parents can be encouraged to introduce such phrase patterns deliberately into daily events with children who are ready for this stage.

Development of symbolic understanding

The stage of pre-language described above usually occurs between eight and twelve months, after which symbolic understanding gradually begins to develop. The first stage is that of object recognition. At about twelve months babies can generalize the idea of a particular object in a particular situation (for example their own cup at a meal time) to all objects which are perceptually recognizable whatever the situation (for example any real-sized cup in any situation). This stage can be demonstrated by giving the child a cup, spoon or brush, and watching to see if he will use it appropriately. This stage of object recognition immediately precedes the development of early symbolic understanding.

From 14 to 15 months, symbolic understanding begins to develop, with an understanding of increasingly 'arbitrary' symbols—in other words with a gradually decreasing perceptual similarity to the object the symbol represents. At this early stage, children may demonstrate an understanding of large doll-play material, such as any appropriate use of a Wendy House-sized tea set. By 18 to 21 months they can usually demonstrate the appropriate use of small doll-play material, such as putting the doll into a tiny bed of doll's house size, and covering it with a blanket. Between 18 and 24 months comes an understanding of two-dimensional representations, as pictures. This can be demonstrated by getting children to match objects to clear coloured pictures (object to symbol). By 2 to $2\frac{1}{4}$ years most children can match small toys to pictures, demonstrating an ability to match one symbol to another. At a still later stage they can match gestures to pictures. By this time the symbols have become truly arbitrary and some verbal language should have begun.

Development of verbal comprehension

Verbal comprehension is the ability to appreciate the meaning contained in a pattern of verbal symbols. Pre-verbal comprehension, in terms of situational understanding has been discussed above. The beginning of true verbal comprehension comes with the understanding of verbal labels. This develops through the following stages:

(i)   situational understanding of the whole phrase;
(ii) situational understanding of labels within the phrase, e.g. 'it's *bed*-time now, here's your *bed*';
(iii) understanding of labels related to objects wherever those objects may be, and no longer linked to a specific phrase pattern, e.g. 'where's your bed?'

At this stage children can select a particular object in response to naming. This is followed by the ability to select a symbolic representation (toy or picture) in response to naming.

The next stage is relating two named objects, such as 'put the *brush* in the *box*'. This usually occurs at about the same stage at which the ability to match symbol to symbol (picture-toy matching) occurs, at 2 to $2\frac{1}{4}$ years.

At a slightly later stage verbal understanding moves from the simple naming of objects to a more indirect verbal relationship such as selecting objects by use, for example 'which one do we cook with?' This stage is reached by most $2\frac{1}{2}$-year-old children. More complex directions, including the use of abstractions such as colour, size, prepositions and negatives can usually be followed by children aged 3 to 4 years, depending, of course, on the complexity of the directions and the number of 'operative' words per sentence.

Development of expressive language

The stages in the development of expressive verbal language follow those of verbal comprehension, but a few months later, in normal development. In the early stages of naming, the attachment of the label to the object is precarious and may depend on a back-up of situational clues, so that a child can name the object when it is in the usual place, but not necessarily in a test situation. It should not be assumed that this failure to name an object during testing is due to inhibition, although it may be, it can also indicate this stage of precarious object-label attachment. Parents may report, for example, that their child can name his cup on the table at home, and are disappointed when this cannot be repeated in a test situation. This stage of precarious label attachment persists in some types of language disorder as a 'word finding' difficulty. Such children may produce words with relative ease in their free play, or in spontaneous conversation, but have difficulty in producing a particular word on request.

By 2 years of age most children are able to produce words other than simple object naming, and many are using three word sentences, often including prepositions. Appropriate use of pronouns comes a little later, at about $2\frac{1}{2}$ years. Most children are reasonably fluent in everyday conversation by about 4 years.

The evolution of sentence forms will not be described in any more detail here, as this has been fully covered by extensive literature already available.

The progression, from the point of view of recovery from a language delay, is the appearance of words and sentences, followed later by the right coding of sounds in words, so early words and phrases may only be understood in context.

Development of intellectual use of language

From the age of about $3\frac{1}{2}$ years verbal language has an increasingly important intellectual function in directing and integrating practical activities, and subsequently becomes internalized as a vehicle for thought. The early stages in this development have been demonstrated experimentally by Luria (1961), and his findings substantiated by other workers. In the early stages of symbolic understanding, any attempt to integrate language into a child's activities is merely disrupting, and he either has to ignore it or forget about whatever he is doing. At the second stage he can be helped by verbal guidance from an adult. By about $3\frac{1}{2}$ years he can take over this role of verbal guidance for himself, and he directs his activities aloud. This is the typical nursery-school stage when children are talking as they play, not necessarily in conversation with others, but rather to help their own play activities. By 4 to 5 years this verbal guidance is usually internalized so that children no longer need to talk aloud in directing, integrating and monitoring their activities, unless the task is very demanding.

The child's own directive-integrative use of language develops in the following way. Quite young children, in the early stages of labelling objects, will attempt to stabilize their own object concepts by naming objects as they handle them. They accompany their play with appropriate noises (e.g. car noises), and later by an abbreviated commentary, which adds an extra dimension to the play and consolidates the ideas they are working out. Language is beginning to integrate different aspects of their activities. Later still, at about $3\frac{1}{2}$ years of age, language immediately precedes the action, so that it is now becoming part of the planning and directing aspect of thinking. The development of this aspect of the intellectual function of language is an important consideration in the developmental language programme, and ways of helping this process in language-handicapped children are described in later chapters. The directive function of language is finally internalized as verbal thinking. As maturation proceeds, the interval of time between planning and action may be lengthened, and eventually the concrete material may be dispensed with so that internalized planning may take over the role of trial and error with concrete material. This final stage does not occur until well into school age, but handicapped children need help so that the foundation stages for this are not held back.

Summary of developmental stages

Figure 1 shows how some of the processes of language development evolve and become interrelated as development proceeds. It shows the central 'pacing' by the intellectual processes of concept formation, and symbolic understanding. Receptive and expressive aspects of verbal language develop from situational understanding to true language when symbolic understanding is established. The whole then becomes integrated as an intellectual process.

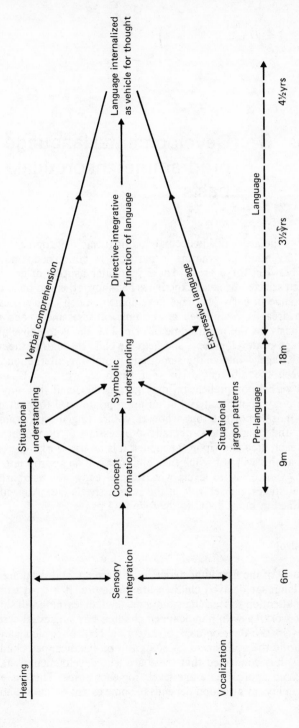

Figure 1 Illustrating the integration of some processes involved in the development of verbal language

Chapter 3 Developmental language programme: theoretical basis

Figure 2 shows the areas of intellectual and linguistic development with which the intervention programme is particularly concerned, and the relationships between these areas. These particular aspects of development have been selected because experience has shown them to be of particular importance in early language development. Each child's present level, in each area, is established at the time of assessment, and this becomes the basis for the programme of help. The aim is to consolidate the present stage of development, and help the child through to the next developmental stage, while at the same time promoting interaction and balance between the different areas. For example, work on listening attention and verbal comprehension may go together, and this may include the use of symbolic material at an appropriate level for that particular child. It is important that whoever is directing the programme should really understand the order and progression of developmental stages within each area shown on the model. It is no use working several stages ahead, as this will not reach the child; nor is it an appropriate use of the time to work only at levels which are already well established. Developmental stages are set out on the record sheets (see Appendix), and are explained in more detail in the following pages.

Attention control

This is obviously of the first importance in all learning, and is an area in which many language-delayed children are immature. If a child cannot give adequate attention to learning situations, then all learning will suffer. Experience of working with handicapped children has suggested certain definite stages in the development of attention control, which can be recognized during the assessment. A study of non-handicapped children (Reynell 1977) has confirmed that these are true developmental stages and has indicated approximate age levels for each stage. There is considerable variability, as attention depends to some extent on the situation,

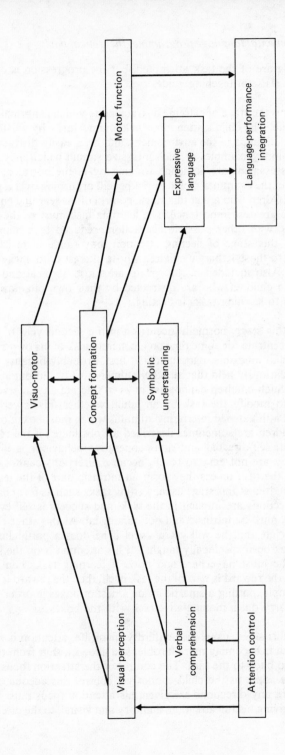

Figure 2 Model used as a basis for language intervention programme

and on the nature of the task attempted, but the progression is definite enough to be a useful teaching guide.

Stage 1: This is the stage of extreme distractability which is normal in the first year of life. The child's attention is held momentarily by whatever is the dominant stimulus in the environment, and he is easily distracted by any new stimulus. Examples of such intrusive stimuli which may occur during the assessment are someone walking by in the corridor; a car hooter outside; the examiner picking up a pencil, or turning over a paper. In teaching children who are at this stage, control of the learning environment is of the greatest importance. The learning task must be the dominant stimulus, with other possible distractions reduced to a minimum. Behaviour at this stage of fleeting attention may range from extreme hyperactivity to those lethargic children whose interest drifts away every few seconds. Also included in this group are those atypical and often very disturbed children who are distracted by their own phantasies, so that attention to learning tasks is fleeting.

Stage 2: At this stage, normally occurring in the second year of life, a child can concentrate for some time on a concrete task of his own choice. This is rigid and inflexible, particularly at first, probably because attention is so precariously held that all other stimuli must be cut out in order to sustain it. Such children cannot use or even tolerate any intervention or attempts to modify the task by an adult, whether this is verbal or visual. This is a threatened interfering stimulus which must be cut out. At this stage children are sometimes described as 'obstinate', if the reasons for their rigid, self-directed and non-cooperative behaviour is not understood. They are not easy to teach, because directions cannot be integrated with the task unless they form an intrinsic part of the learning task itself. Children at this stage usually enjoy tasks such as form boards, where the directions are implicit in the task, and success is self-evident. Rewards, too, must be intrinsic and not contingent. At this stage a child can. it appreciate that he will get a sweet if he does a particular task (unless this has been specifically taught). If his attention is on the sweet, this is what he must have here and now. If learning tasks can be so arranged that the reward is part of the task itself, then the reward is effective. For example, putting a smartie inside a nest of boxes in order to get the child to carry out a manipulative task with the boxes.

Stage 3: At this stage, usual in the third year of life, attention is single-channelled, but is becoming more flexible, and allows a shift from task to directions, and back to the task. The control of the attention focus is entirely with the adult, as the child cannot yet control this adequately for himself. Before any directions are given, his attention focus must be set so that he is giving his full attention, auditory and visual, to the directions which are to be given. He then needs help in transferring the directions immediately to the task. In teaching situations it is important to make sure the child is sitting still, without fiddling with the toys or other teaching material, and that he is looking at the speaker's face if the directions are verbal. He can only assimilate directions if his whole attention is on the source from which they come, whether this is verbal or a demonstration.

Stage 4: During the fourth year of life most children can begin to control their own attention focus. Attention is still single-channelled, so that a child must give his full attention, visual and auditory, to any directions being given to him, but he does this spontaneously and under his own control, without needing to have his attention focus set by an adult before each verbal direction is given. He moves gradually towards a stage where he only needs to look at the speaker when the directions become difficult for him to understand.

Stage 5: This is the stage of school readiness where a child can assimilate verbal directions related to the task he is engaged upon, without needing to interrupt the task and look at the speaker. This two-channelled attention, integrating auditory and visual (or manipulatory) learning, is at first sustained only for short periods, after which the interest of one or other aspect takes over. When children have reached this stage of attention control they are ready for teaching in a class, where directions are often given to the class as a whole while the children are carrying out a task.

Stage 6: This is a mature school entry level where integrated attention is well established and well sustained.

Concept formation

Concept formation begins with the awareness of permanence of objects, which can usually be demonstrated by the age of 9 or 10 months. Until this stage all thinking is dependent on immediate perception. Children who come into the language programmes are usually well beyond this stage of concept formation, because it is not possible to diagnose a specific language delay as early as this. They are usually ready to understand simple abstract components, such as colour and shape, at the level of perceptual matching, so the stages set out on the schedules start at this level.

(1) *One-to-one matching:* This involves simple concrete matching according to one abstract component at a time, starting with similar objects (e.g. red brick to red brick, and blue brick to blue brick) so that there are no other distracting variables. When varied objects can be matched ac-

cording to colour (e.g. red ball to red brick) the concept of colour, as an abstraction, is understood. The same holds for shape matching (round to round; square to square, etc.). Later on, children can form more advanced concepts by integrating more than one abstract component at a time.

(2) *Classification:* By this stage the children have really understood the simple abstract components and can classify a variety of objects according to one abstract dimension at a time, e.g. classifying according to colour, shape, type of object, and later according to use (e.g. all things used for dressing, for eating, for the garden, etc.).

(3) *Size and quantity:* These abstractions are a little more difficult to understand than are colour and shape. The first understanding is of two simple categories such as big/small; or long/short. This can be demonstrated, as with colour and shape, by simple one-to-one matching, and later by sorting into two categories. When this is really understood, sorting can lead on to grading, using more than one category at a time, e.g. size ordering. Understanding of quantity comes later than understanding of size. The concepts of 'more' and 'less' are understood before the concept of 'same', which comes surprisingly late. 'Same' and 'different', and 'like' and 'unlike' need to be taught not only in terms of quantity, but also with other components, so that children learn to select which one is 'not the same as the others'. With language-retarded children this may need to be taught non-verbally at first so that their language difficulty does not interfere, perhaps using a hand sign to 'label' the concept. This is explained further in chapter 5.

(4) *Positional concepts:* The very early understanding of 'in and out' at a purely perceptual level begins soon after 12 months when children put objects into containers, but it is not until much later that positions are understood as abstractions, at the level of concepts rather than percepts. The order in which the positional concepts are set out on the schedule has been found by experience to be the most usual order for development, and is therefore a rational one for teaching.

Symbolic understanding

The developmental progression of symbolic understanding has been explained in chapter 2. The stages set out on the schedule for teaching follow this progression, and are explained here in a little more detail.

(1) *Object recognition:* At this stage a child has a few object-concepts such that object recognition is no longer dependent on exactly similar

perceptual components, and situational clues. He will recognize everyday objects such as a brush, spoon or cup, in any place at any time, even if it is slightly different from the one he uses at home. These must first of all be the right size, but later can be recognized even if reduced to a smaller size.

(2) *Large doll-play:* Doll-play is a useful way of assessing and teaching early symbols, as the materials are closely related to everyday living, and can represent those used at the object recognition stage. The early stages of doll-play are demonstrated by an appropriate relationship of two components, such as putting the spoon in the cup, or brushing the doll's hair. Later on sequences can be acted out, such as making tea and handing round cups, using a tea-set of Wendy House-size. This is truly representational play, using easy symbols which are perceptually still fairly similar to the real objects. At first the children may only be able to understand this sort of play alongside their own activity, such as feeding the doll at their own mealtimes, or bathing the doll while having their own bath. A child may also need adult modelling, to demonstrate the play sequence first. When he has really established some understanding of these play sequences for himself, he is ready to go on to the stage of small doll-play.

(3) *Small doll-play:* When children can understand these small toys, they have reached a stage of understanding symbols which may be perceptually very different from the objects they represent. Again the early stages are simple relationships of two components, leading later to playing out sequences. Home scenes are the easiest to understand, but small boys may prefer to use cars, roads and garages, or perhaps farm animals. Village play is the most advanced form of play with this small three-dimensional material. This involves an understanding which goes beyond the immediate home environment extending the boundaries to an understanding of symbolic representations of streets, shops, and parks, etc. Few children under the age of 4 years can manage this level of village play, but for children of upper-nursery or infant-school level who have difficulty with language, it can be a useful alternative form of expression.

(4) *Role playing:* This does not fit easily into a symbolic sequence as it is qualitatively somewhat different, and is very variable from one child to another. Some children have a greater need for this sort of 'pretend' play than others, but most children enjoy dressing up, playing buses, or playing 'house'. The material used for this sort of play may vary from real objects to something which is truly arbitrary, or even purely imaginative, such as an imaginary companion.

(5) *Two-dimensional symbols:* Recognition of two-dimensional symbols

(pictures) usually comes before the stage of acting out meaningful sequences with the small toys, but later than the ability to recognize and relate small toys meaningfully. In other words there is a considerable overlap in the stages of symbol recognition, and the use of these symbols as a medium for expression. It cannot be assumed that a recognition of pictures implies an ability to play freely with small toys. The ability to match an object to a picture leads on to the ability to match a toy to a picture. This is an important stage indicating the ability to relate one type of symbol to another. This ability is basic to verbal language conversation (translating a receptive verbal symbol pattern into an expressive verbal symbol response) and so is an important teaching stage for language-delayed children.

(6) *Gestures:* The understanding and use of gestures, and later even perhaps more abstract hand signs, may be important for children who are very delayed in verbal language development. Learning to make the appropriate gesture for a particular picture, or to select a picture in response to a gesture, can be a useful way through to verbal language for some children. Training at this level of symbolic understanding is not usually necessary if children have already developed verbal language.

Verbal comprehension

The stages in pre-verbal comprehension have been described in chapter 2. Situational understanding of familiar phrases precedes the development of symbolic understanding. True verbal comprehension, as representative language, begins with the understanding of verbal labels. This is, of course, dependent on, and an aspect of, symbolic understanding. The verbal comprehension schedules begin at this stage of understanding verbal labels, but some children may need plenty of work on non-verbal symbols before they are ready even for this level of teaching. The developmental progression of verbal comprehension has been described briefly in chapter 2. A more detailed description of the teaching stages on the schedule is as follows:

(1) *Verbal labels:* As with any true symbol, verbal labels can represent the named object at any time and in any place, and can be applied to any object of similar class. For example the word 'cup' applies to any cup, in any situation. The words 'milk' or 'drink' applied to the object cup are not true verbal labels as they are situationally linked words. At first the word will only have meaning in the presence of the object. In the very early learning stage, the word will need to be supplied while the child is actually handling and using the object, e.g. 'brush', as he handles the brush and brushes his hair. This moves on to the stage at which he can hand a named object on request, from a choice of two or three objects.

Only if this is reliable and repeatable in different situations can
labels be considered really established.

(2) *Relating two named objects:* The stages of verbal understanding,
which have been selected for teaching and recording, follow the development of the understanding of concepts. Still at the stage of object-
concepts, a child may be able to assimilate two at a time before he can
understand words such as verbs and adjectives which imply a higher level
of conceptual understanding. For this reason the stage of 'noun-noun'
links follows the stage of understanding single verbal labels and precedes
the more linguistically rational 'noun-verb' sentences. Understanding of
qualifying words such as adjectives must await the understanding of the
relevant abstraction, e.g. 'big', 'red', 'more', etc. If the word is taught
before the concept is understood, it will tend to become situationally
linked (e.g. 'little', only applied to 'little boy'). It is appropriate to teach
the word and the concept together, as one reinforces the other. When a
child can follow directions containing three or more operative words, and
can do this reliably for all the words in his vocabulary, he is near to
school readiness in verbal understanding.

Expressive language

The stages followed in the developmental programme for expressive
language are the same as those described for verbal comprehension, but
occur a little later, so no further description will be given here. For a
more detailed study of the evolution of expressive language, the reader is
referred to the extensive literature on linguistics.

Intellectual use of language (the directive-integrative function)

The schedules include stages in two aspects of language use:

  (i) language as communication, and
  (ii) language as an intellectual process in planning, guiding and integrating practical activities.

Language as communication is self-explanatory on the record sheet, so
needs no further amplification.
   The programme follows the developmental stages first established
experimentally by Luria (1961) and subsequently confirmed by others. In
the developmental programme, verbal language as a symbol system is all
important, whereas in Luria's experiments it was nearer to a signal
system. The use of language in planning, directing and integrating practical activities depends on formulating the directions verbally, first aloud,
and then as the internalized language of thought. This gives a new dimension to thinking, allowing actions to be pre-planned and organized so that

this does not need to depend on actual trial and error, and eventually can be carried out in the absence of the concrete material. It is this important intellectual function of language which is the ultimate aim in helping pre-school children who have delayed language development, so that they are not denied this intellectual process at the stage of development at which it becomes important. The stages set out for teaching and recording are as follows:

(1) *Pre-integration:* At this early stage, when language is just begin-ning to develop, it needs all the child's attention, so he is not able to relate verbal directions to any action he is carrying out. Any attempt to in-troduce verbal directions, while he is carrying out a task, must either be ignored, or disrupt the task. This is close to Stage (2) in attention control (see above), and developmentally related to it, in normal development. In language-delayed children it is possible for visual directions to be in-tegrated at higher levels of attention, while verbal directions still interfere. In teaching children at this stage of language use, the language must be very simple, have a direct and immediate concrete referent, and back up, rather than replace visual directions. For example, 'the brick goes on top', while showing or helping the child to do this. Care should be taken not to over-verbalize at this stage or the child may form a habit of cutting out verbal directions. For example, a four-year-old, while playing well with small toys, had to stop and cover her ears with her hands to cut out per-sistent interfering verbal directions from her father.

(2) *Adult verbalization helps:* At this stage an adult can help a child to carry out a concrete task by introducing very simple verbal directions. The directions must be immediately related to the task, but can now preceed the action instead of accompanying it, as in teaching at stage one. Verbalization can become truly directive, e.g. 'Put another one on top' may enable a child to make a block bridge which he could not do without the verbal direction. Language is beginning to be used as an in-tellectual process to help solve practical problems, but at this stage the language must be supplied by the adult, as the child cannot yet do this for himself.

(3) *Child externalizes language:* At this third developmental stage the child can begin to direct and integrate his own actions by talking aloud. At first his language is just an accompaniment to his play, but gradually it becomes more than this, and he can be heard giving himself simple directions immediately preceding the action, so helping to plan it. Children who are already attempting this intellectual use of language, but who still have very little verbal language available to them, are in great need of help with language development so that they may achieve this im-portant intellectual integration. This sort of self-monitoring depends on

actually formulating the directions and saying them aloud, so that a child can use this verbal planning and his own auditory feed-back.

At first this is very deliberate and slow, but later becomes a more natural process and he begins to internalize part of the directions, or to reduce his self-monitoring to a whisper.

(4) *Language internalized:* By this stage self-monitoring by verbal direction has become so much part of the intellectual make-up that directions need not be said aloud. The use made of externalized language may continue for specially difficult tasks, but directive language is internalized for simple tasks so integration does not have to wait upon the actual speaking of the words. Finally an abbreviated symbol system may be used as internalized language in thinking.

At all stages, particularly the last two, levels of function will vary according to the situation and the difficulty of the tasks, which will need to be borne in mind in teaching and in assessing the stage reached. Even some mature adults revert to externalized language direction when working out a particularly difficult problem.

The record sheets allow for separate recording of the use of language in concrete intellectual tasks and in free play.

Performance abilities, non-linguistic

Performance abilities include non-verbal concrete tasks such as form boards and picture puzzles (visual perceptual); copying models (visuomotor); and creative building. By definition, most of the children coming into developmental language programmes have better performance than linguistic abilities, so these areas may need less direct work on them. However, as the understanding of concrete material helps to build up basic concepts, which in turn are fundamental to language development, these performance areas must play an integral part in any language programme for pre-school children. It is therefore important for whoever is directing the programme to be aware of the developmental progression in visual perception, visuo-motor understanding, and motor creative abilities, and to understand how these developmental areas are related to language (see Figure 2).

(1) *Visual perception:* A task is considered to be mainly visual perceptual when its solution depends on simple visual matching, with minimal need for higher intellectual processes such as abstraction or more complex relationships. These higher levels, or more 'central' aspects, are included under the heading of concept formation. One-to-one matching, as described in the early stages of concept formation, is usually mainly a visual perceptual match using one dimension, such as fitting shapes to in-

sets in a form board; or pointing to a shape or colour that matches the 'master' shape or colour used in teaching or testing. Visual perception of this sort requires a relatively superficial aspect of intellectual processing. Many mentally handicapped children can achieve spuriously high scores on the form-board type of test, but without the backing of concept formation at the higher processing levels, so it is important to see that the teaching of concepts goes along with that of visual perception. In other words, there is a limit to the intellectual help children can get from endless practice at jigsaws and visual perceptual tasks of that sort.

As soon as possible children should be moved on from simple shape matching to more constructional three-dimensional tasks, such as those included under the headings of visuo-motor and motor-creative.

(2) *Visuo-motor and constructional tasks:* Visuo-motor tasks involve the visual perception of a two or three dimensional model, and the reconstruction of the model either directly or from memory, e.g. copying a block bridge. This is a more complex task than simple perceptual matching as the child has to assimilate the model, and recreate a 'match' using a different modality (motor organization). A higher level still is the ability to create a model from an inner concept, for example putting together a wooden manikin from his internalized concept of a person, where there is no model to copy (Reynell 1970).

The stages used in sampling these abilities for the purpose of teaching and recording progress are set out on the schedules. The order in which they appear has been found by experience to be the appropriate developmental sequence. The methods of teaching, and assessment of the stages achieved, are described in chapter 5.

Chapter 4   Assessment and establishment of programme basis

A very full assessment of children's abilities and handicaps is essential in order to establish a programme basis, and to see whether the children are suitable for this type of programme (see chapter 1). This should include paediatric assessment, hearing tests, social assessment, and if necessary psychiatric investigations. Psychological and linguistic assessments form the actual basis of the programme, so these will be discussed in more detail than the other aspects.

(1) Paediatric assessment

It is not appropriate here to discuss this aspect in any detail. The purpose of this volume is to guide those who are directing the language programme, and clearly a paediatric assessment needs very specialized knowledge. A professional person directing the language programme (such as a speech therapist or teacher) should have access to at least a summary of the paediatric report. Severe language delay may well be the presenting feature of a more extensive handicapping condition which needs both other forms of help and some understanding of the total situation by whoever undertakes to help the child's language development. Ideally this information is obtained by personal contact and discussion with the paediatrician or medical officer, so that the full implications with regard to helping language development are understood. Every effort should be made to develop this direct liaison, but if it is not possible, there should at least be access to a report of any relevant factors. The reporting needs to be mutual and continued, so that not only may the programme director be aware of the implications of the handicap as far as language development is concerned, but also that the paediatrician or medical officer may be aware of the child's response to the help provided.

(2) Hearing tests

Any child who has a language delay needs very careful hearing tests. Screening tests are not enough. Several of the children in the Wolfson

Centre study had minor degrees of hearing impairment, usually intermittent, but enough to contribute materially to their difficulty in learning language. If a child has a primary language disability, any situation which makes language learning more difficult, such as intermittent ear infections, needs specially careful investigation so that appropriate remedial measures may be taken to remove or minimize this contributory problem. Where there is any question of a hearing difficulty, however minor or transient, hearing tests should be repeated regularly.

(3) Social assessment

As the Wolfson Centre study was concerned with children suffering from a constitutionally determined central language delay or disorder (see chapter 1), it included no children for whom the social environment was considered to be the primary or sole cause of the language delay. In many cases, however, there may be very considerable social contributing factors, which need careful assessment. Also, it is important to be fully aware of the social assets and limitations within which they are working. Social assessment is to some extent a specialized field, so no full description is attempted in this volume.

(4) Psychiatric assessment

No children presenting with primary psychiatric disorders were included in the Wolfson Centre study, for the reason stated above, but in a few cases problems were complicated by psychiatric factors to an extent which necessitated seeking specialist advice.

(5) Psychological assessment

A conventional psychological assessment in the form of an 'intelligence test' is not appropriate when the purpose is to plan a programme of help for a language-handicapped child. Assessment needs to be in terms of a breakdown into different areas of intellectual function, and an assessment of the level and pattern of learning in whatever areas are selected as important. The areas shown in Figure 2, and described in chapter 3, have been found to be important for language development. Assessment of these areas forms the basis of the developmental programme. Assessment of each area separately would take a long time, and more sustained concentration than these young children are able to give, so the examiner needs to be constantly aware of the total framework he is assessing, and must use every piece of observed behaviour and test response to contribute towards this. An outline of the procedure follows, but the way in which this is carried out must depend very much on the child. With some highly deviant and uncooperative children much of the assessment is by structured observation (Reynell, 1970).

(a) *Attention control*

This can be observed from the child's response to any tests which require attention focus, and from the amount of control the examiner needs to exert. The attention stages, and the indicative behaviour patterns, are fully described in chapter 3. To some extent this amounts to a subjective judgement, and is only partly quantifiable, but experience has shown reasonably close agreement between different examiners.

(b) *Symbolic understanding*

A standardized test has recently been produced by Lowe (1975), which will give an age level for symbolic understanding in relation to small toys. In the absence of a sophisticated test scale such as this, a teaching level, and approximate age equivalent can be obtained by the following procedure:

(i) *Object recognition:* (12 to 14 months). Put a brush, cup, spoon and toothbrush in front of the child and see whether he will use any of them appropriately or demonstrate any meaningful relationship between them.

(ii) *Large doll-play:* (15 to 18 months). Using material of Wendy House-size, put a doll, cup, brush and spoon on the table and see whether the child uses any of the toys appropriately, relates them meaningfully, or carries out any play sequences. If he does not appear to recognize the toys, demonstrate some simple relationship such as brushing the doll's hair or giving the doll a drink, and see whether the child will imitate this. If this adult modelling leads to meaningful play on the child's part, this is an indication that he is ready for teaching at this level.

(iii) *Small doll-play:* (18 to 21 months). The above procedure is repeated using doll's house-sized toys. A small doll, bed and blanket is enough to start with. If this is meaningful to the child, produce further toys such as a table and chair or bath, to see whether he is ready for playing out sequences. His response to the play material, with and without adult modelling, will indicate the teaching level for which he is ready.

(iv) *Picture/object matching:* (22 to 24 months). Very clear coloured photographs should be used, depicting just one familiar object against a blank background, such as those in the Ladybird Picture series. Four pictures, pasted on postcards, are placed in front of the child. He is then given matching objects one at a time, to see whether he can match the object to the picture. The objects should be 'real' size, not toys, at this stage, as he may only be able to manage one symbol at a time. Also the objects should be perceptually a little different from the picture so that it is the object concept which determines the match, and not a superficial attribute such as colour. For example, if the picture shows a pink brush, match this with a white object-brush. It will be necessary to demonstrate the first one to give the child the idea of what is required.

(v) *Picture/toy matching:* (24 to 26 months). The same procedure is carried out, using small toys instead of real objects to match to the pictures (see Plate 1). This will demonstrate the child's ability to match one type of symbol to another.

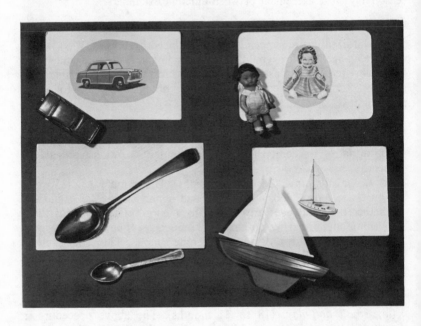

(vi) *Gesture/picture matching:* (2½+ years). Select four clear pictures which will allow a simple gesture match, such as a bed (sleep gesture), car (driving gesture), and cup (drinking gesture). This is equivalent to a non-verbal selection by use (noun-verb), and so is considerably more difficult than the non-verbal object-symbol stages above. This stage of understanding can have a receptive and expressive aspect. First see whether the child can select the appropriate picture in response to a gesture. Then see whether he can give the appropriate gesture in response to pointing to the picture. It is best to use the same set of pictures at first so that he knows what is wanted, but vary the order of presentation. This will demonstrate a teaching level with regard to the use of a non-verbal language system for children who have such severe verbal language difficulties that they need hand signs as a way through.

(vii) *Village-play:* As explained in chapter 3, this is a relatively advanced type of symbolic play, not usually encountered before 4 years of age. It is useful to assess the readiness for this sort of play with children who have a limited ability for verbal expression, as it is an alternative form of language expression. Leave the child to play freely with the material and see whether he merely classifies the toys (lining up houses, trees, etc.) or whether he is able to develop this into an imaginative play sequence.

(c) *Concept formation*

A qualitative assessment can be carried out by sampling the developmental stages described in chapter 3. This will give a useful teaching basis even if no age equivalent is available. In order to get an age level for this area of development, standardized tests are needed. There are very few uncontaminated tests of concept formation available, although most general intelligence scales contain some items which come near to this. Francis-Williams (1970) describes a test produced by Frances Graham which gives approximate age levels. This is a sorting task, using blocks which vary according to the dimensions of shape, colour and size. The level of success depends on the use and integration of these dimensions in sorting the material. In the Wolfson Centre programme a similar type of task was used. This is a matching task using wooden animal forms, which vary according to the three dimensions of colour, topological shape, and shape detail (see Plate 2). There are approximate age norms for this scale over the critical age range of $2\frac{1}{2}$ to 5 years, but it is not yet published.

(d) *Performance, non-linguistic*

As with concept formation, some qualitative assessment may be obtained by sampling the abilities described in chapter 3. Important 'milestones' such as building towers, walls and bridges, can be observed during free play with bricks, or as a more structured test situation in copying models. Most of the standardized tests for performance abilities are designed around these basic developmental stages. The Merrill Palmer, Gesell and Griffiths Scales all include form boards (visual perception), and copying simple models (visuo-motor), with age norms for the specially designed test situation and material. The performance sub-scale of the Griffiths Scale (Griffiths 1970) was the most often used standardized performance scale in the Wolfson Centre study, as this has a relatively recent standardization, and contains a reasonable selection of appropriate performance tests for sampling the type of abilities included in the developmental language programme. The age score represents a composite score for visual-perceptual and visuo-motor tasks, so the examiner needs to look carefully to see whether the balance of achievement is appropriate (see pp. 35–6), or whether nearly all the success depends on the more peripheral

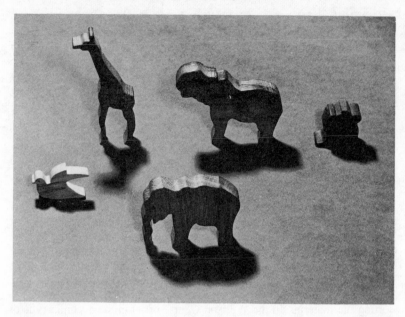

visual perceptual items. The scale includes a useful block design section, which enables rather more central processing to be sampled, and also provides a good opportunity to assess the directive use of language (see below).

(e) *Verbal comprehension and expressive language*

Most of the stages in verbal language, which are relevant to the developmental language programme are fully described in the manual for the RDLS (Reynell, 1969); so only a brief outline of the assessment will be given here. For those who have access to standardized language scales, a quantitative assessment can be obtained for different aspects of verbal language, particularly a separate assessment of receptive and expressive aspects. If this is not available, a teaching basis may be established by sampling the developmental stages described in previous chapters.

(i) *Situational understanding:* The child's mother will be able to report on familiar phrases to which he will respond. These should be demonstrated in the test situation before being recorded as present, e.g. 'do pat-a-cake'.

(ii) A move towards the understanding of verbal labels can be demonstrated by asking for some object the child is reported to know well, e.g. 'Where's Teddy?' At this intermediary stage he may only recognize his own Teddy as a 'Teddy' without any generalization.

(iii) A true understanding of verbal labels is established when he can reliably select a named object in a test situation from a choice of at least three.

(iv) *Relating two named objects:* Ask the child to relate two named objects, from a choice of not less than four. He must assimilate both verbal labels before picking up one of the objects, to be sure he has achieved this stage, e.g. the directive 'put the *brush* in the *box*' must be complete before he picks up the brush or handles the box.

(v) Understanding of noun-verb links, and more complex sentences can be demonstrated using pictures or toys, with a reasonable selection to ensure that it is the response to the verbal direction, and not to the other clues, which determines the action, e.g. 'Show me the girl sitting on a chair', could be achieved just by understanding verbal labels if there is only one girl to choose from. This could be very misleading in terms of the child's level of understanding.

Similar stages for expressive language can be assessed by eliciting words and phrases in carefully structured situations with toys and pictures.

(f) *Intellectual use of language*

The use of language as a directive-integrative function can be assessed by observation during performance tests and during free play with symbolic toys. The stages for assessment, and the behaviour which indicates these, are fully described in chapter 3. There is no need to devise specific test situations to elicit this aspect of development. Provided the examiner has a clear understanding of the stages as described, the child's level will become clear from observation.

(g) *Articulation and linguistic structure*

Although these aspects of speech and language are important for older children, particularly those with very specific types of language disorder, they are not particularly relevant to the developmental language programme. The children who can be helped by the developmental approach described here have too little central language ability for more detailed work on these specific aspects. When there was enough expressive language, articulation was regularly assessed in the Wolfson Centre study, but the findings did not play a major part in planning a programme of help, as this was concerned with central language. When the central (cognitive) aspects of language are fully resolved, a different approach may be appropriate to work on any remaining difficulties with specific speech sounds or linguistic structuring (see chapter 1).

Chapter 5 Planning and carrying out the developmental language programme

Introduction

The actual carrying out of the programmes is described in this chapter in general terms. Further details are expanded in the case studies described in chapter 6. The basic procedures are the same for 'parent' and 'class' situations, although the actual setting is different. The descriptions of teaching the different intellectual and linguistic processes described in previous chapters are combined for the two different settings. The main difference is that in the 'parent' programme it is the parents who carry out the day to day education under the direction of the speech therapist; whereas in the 'class' programme the teacher is both directing and carrying out the teaching herself. The actual teaching, whether carried out by parents in the home, or by the teacher in the class, is very similar. In each case the child's individual programme is followed, using whatever situations and materials are appropriate to the particular setting.

Description of setting for parent programme and class programme

Parent programme

By using parents as teachers and adapting the home environment to the child's level of understanding and learning needs, it is possible to help children over a wider age range than in a class. In the class they need to be old enough to tolerate separation from their parents, and to be able to adapt to a small group. Children may start in the 'parent' programme from the age of 2 years. This is really the earliest age at which it is possible to recognize a specific language handicap, although a generalized intellectual delay may be evident much earlier. Findings so far have indicated that the younger the child the better the progress, so children are taken on for help as soon as a language handicap is recognized.

The need for this help is recognized at assessment, and referral made to the speech therapist who then arranges regular visits with the parents. The speech therapy sessions are aimed at showing the parents how to communicate with the child, and how to bring language learning into daily living, so this is an intensive and ongoing learning experience adapted to his particular needs. Even very busy mothers who may have several children and go out to work, can still use the daily bathing, feeding and dressing times to help their child's language development, if they have guidance on how best to use these times. One, or both, parents are seen with the child once in six weeks. Experience has shown this to be the most effective interval of time in most cases. It allows enough time for some progress to have been made, so that further advice can be given in helping the child on to the next stage of development. A few parents have needed more frequent visits at first, but as soon as possible it is advisable to increase the interval to once in six weeks. Among the reasons for reducing the sessions to once in six weeks are:

(1) It is realistic in terms of the child's developmental needs to expect significant progress in this period. If the visits are too frequent, therapists can only repeat advice previously given, which is not a very rewarding situation.

(2) Most people are short of time, so it is wise to be economical with the speech therapist's and the parents' time so that this may be used to the best advantage for the children. The six-weekly sessions enable the child to have a very intensive programme at home, while conserving the time spent travelling to and from the clinic. It also allows the speech therapist to see more children than she could if each child had a weekly appointment.

(3) In the Wolfson Centre study the attendance rate was very high indeed (over 90 per cent), which is not the case when parents are expected to bring their children every week.

(4) Finally, and less often recognized, is the need to avoid over-involvement in the personal problems of the parents. It is not the role of the speech therapist to become a psycho-therapist for the parents. This needs skills in which they are not trained. Clearly this sort of support cannot be avoided altogether, nor should it be, but it is too easy for parents to use a weekly session for working out their own personal problems with the therapist, and using the therapist as a 'leaning post', rather than focusing on the child and themselves becoming a support for the child. This sort of over-dependence can be avoided if the appointments are only once in six weeks.

It may be either or both parents who attend with the child, or in some cases a grandparent. It should be someone who takes on much of the day to day management of the child, so that the home programme can be realistic and regularly carried out.

Experience has shown that parents are better able to understand the procedures if these are demonstrated during the session rather than just explained. The session, therefore, takes the form of a demonstration of situations which occur in daily living, which can be used as language learning experiences, such as feeding and dressing. This may be carried out in 'real' situations, or with dolls, if the child is ready for this sort of symbolic understanding. Parents can then take over during the session, and carry on the situation with the child, so that the therapist can see that the demonstration and advice have been understood. In this way modifications in handling and communication can be understood in a very practical way in relation to everyday living. Each session becomes a three-way involvement with parent, child and therapist, rather than just the therapist giving advice. This is in contrast to the more traditional type of speech therapy in which the therapist sees the child alone, and then gives the parents 'homework'.

Each session lasts approximately an hour to an hour and a half, and includes taking the family down to the waiting room for coffee and orange juice, putting coats on and toiletting. This is all part of the practical situation which is used for creating an appropriate language-learning environment.

Children can be accepted into the 'parent' programme from a fairly wide geographical area, as they are only expected to attend once in six weeks; and the programme can be adapted for children with a wide range of handicaps including those who would be difficult to help in a group or class.

Class programme

Class children in the Wolfson Centre study were aged between 3 and 5+ years. They were pre-school classes, so the aim was to get children ready for school by the age of 5 years. The ceiling was slightly elastic, according to the child's needs, but very few children stayed on after the age of $5\frac{1}{2}$ years. Under $3\frac{1}{2}$ years of age most children are not able to adapt to groups without the presence of their parents. A few children between 3 and $3\frac{1}{2}$ years were accepted, usually because there was a sibling in the group.

There were two classes, each of 8 children. Each class met every day during school term, one class in the mornings and one in the afternoons. A few children were tried part time (e.g. one or two mornings a week), but they found it difficult to adapt, and the five day week programme was very much more successful. The morning and afternoon sessions were for two hours, and were very intensive. The number of children was dictated by the size of the room, but if space allows a suitable number would be 10 children to one teacher and nursery assistant.

New children were introduced one at a time, making sure that the group was really stable so that a new child could have the attention he needed without disrupting the group. This is important, as a new child can easily disrupt what has been carefully built up with the other children. Many of these young, language-handicapped children have behaviour difficulties, and are immature in other ways, so it is important that each step achieved should not be undone by the indiscriminate admission of a new child.

Although most of the children came by school transport, with an escort, it was insisted that parents should come with new children, and stay for as long as their child needed this. A careful transfer of dependence was carried out from parent to teacher, usually within the first two or three days. A traumatic and over-quick separation may cause difficulties which delay adjustment and, incidentally, upset the whole group, so it is important that the admission stages are very carefully handled. Ideally work with the parents (as in the 'parent' programme) would be carried out alongside the class programme, so that teaching could be reinforced at home, but staff time does not usually allow this combination. In any case a close link with the parents is essential, so parents were invited sometimes to watch the class and discuss ways of helping the child with the teacher afterwards. However effective the class, it is for only two hours a day, so it is important to have cooperation from the parents at home if the child is to make the fastest possible progress.

In order to make the best possible use of the class session, the teaching should be intensive, so that no time is wasted in activities that are not related to the language-learning needs of the child. Playing on the climbing frame, for example, is of course fun, and may fulfil some physical need, but it can be done at other times of the day when expert teaching help is not available, so it is not an appropriate use of the two-hour class session. Orange juice and biscuit time, on the other hand, lends itself very well to a language learning situation, so can appropriately form part of the daily programme.

Integration into school at the age of 5 years also needs to be carefully handled in order that the improvements effected in the pre-school language class may continue. In the Wolfson Centre study a very close liaison was forged between the teacher of the language class and the teacher of the school to which the child would transfer. This was accomplished by visits to the school by the language-class teacher before transfer, and, when possible, visits to the language class by the teacher of the school. A follow-up visit was always made by the language-class teacher after transfer, so that any difficulties arising after a few weeks could be discussed. For some children it was considered advisable to 'stagger' the transfer, so that for the first term they would continue to attend the language class for half days while attending school also for half days. Local schools were very cooperative in this way, and it proved to be a great help for some of the less mature children. Handled in this way, there were very few transfer problems for any of the children in the study, and nearly all of them continued to make good language progress.

Work on the developmental areas shown in Figure 2

(1) *Attention control*

Many of the children referred for help with language handicaps have very immature attention control, so this is considered to be a very important aspect of the work.

(a) *Stage 1:* The younger children, coming into the parent programme, are often at stages 1 or 2 in attention control (see p. 28). With children showing high distractability (level 1), the teaching is directed towards helping them to focus and hold their attention on anything that interests them, so gradually moving them on to level 2. By observation of the child's free activity, and discussion with the parents, it is possible to find the materials and activities most likely to interest the child. Then a plan for using this material is worked out, so that a short task with quick success is achieved. The task, whether it is listening, or a practical activity, or a combination of the two, must be intrinsically rewarding to the child, so that he sees it as worthwhile to carry through. Once his interest is lost, it is no use at this stage to force it back. It is better to repeat the process with whatever is his next brief interest, quickly turning it into a rewarding exercise. This needs plenty of ingenuity, and parents need to be convinced of its importance if they are to make this effort at home. They need constant reassurance that this work on attention is basic to language development, and that direct work on language will follow later when the child is ready. If they are mainly concerned about the failure to 'talk' they may not immediately see the relevance of work on listening and attention for themselves. The therapist can pick out examples of the child's interests, during the session, and relate these to similar situations which may occur at home, which could be used for sustaining attention. At this stage the teaching situation should be as free as possible from unnecessary distractions, such as constant bombardment of sound from radio and television. By judiciously enhancing the interest of whatever the child chooses to do, and reducing other distractions as far as the situation allows, parents and teachers may structure the environment to help the child. He may, for example, show a momentary interest in the soap at bath time. His mother may be shown how this interest could be sustained by helping him to rub the soap on his skin, and feel the smoothness and pleasant scent it imparts, moving from one part of his body to another. This is better learning for him than quickly moving on to splashing water over him, which only acts as another distraction.

(b) *Stage 2:* This is the stage at which the child's attention is held rigidly and inflexibly by whatever he decides to do. He cannot integrate, or even tolerate any sort of adult participation. Successful teaching depends on the therapist, parent or teacher making the directions and reward become part of the task itself, so that learning can be achieved despite the child's inability to integrate to an adult's attempt to modify the task. Directions at first need to go alongside the task, as an incidental accompaniment. For example, if the child is building a single straight tower, the teacher may sit beside him and build herself a double tower, without actually interfering with the child's own construction; or a verbal commentary may be introduced such as 'one brick, another brick, and another one on top'. This may gradually help him to integrate other aspects of his own task without a direct attempt to modify it, which he could not yet accept. Children at this stage of attention control may be seen in class as 'good' children who will concentrate for a long time, but close observation shows the activities to be repetitive and rigid, which actually blocks further learning unless help is given in the ways suggested above. All adaptations must be with the adult at first. The adult must become part of the task, and only very gradually introduce slight modifications by allowing the directions (verbal or visual) to go a little ahead instead of the earlier stage of going alongside the task. When the child can adapt to this he is moving towards stage 3.

(c) *Stage 3:* This is a slightly easier teaching stage, but still one at which the adult needs to be very much in control. To make the most of the emerging ability to adapt to directions, the child needs constant help in transferring the focus of his attention, as explained in chapter 3. Parents and teachers need to be aware of the part they can play at this stage. Two examples will illustrate this:

(i) Towards the end of a session with the speech therapist, James was standing looking out of the window watching children in the playground. His mother said to him, 'Do you want an orange juice?' James appeared not to have heard this as his visual attention was fully absorbed elsewhere, and nobody had helped him to switch the focus to listening to his mother. The therapist then went up to him, turned him round to face her, and then said 'Do you want an orange juice?' The message was immediately understood as the speaker now had his full and undivided attention, and the response was very positive. This made a good teaching example for the mother, as to how to help his attention focus at home.

(ii) In the classroom Janet was playing in the sand. An adult passed and said 'Make me a castle'. Janet took no notice. The teacher then went up to Janet, turned her face round so that she could see the teacher's face, and gently prevented her hands from fiddling with the sand. Then when she had Janet's full attention the teacher said 'Make me a castle.' The teacher helped her to transfer her attention focus immediately back to the sand so that Janet was able to understand and respond to the request.

If this sort of training is to be effective, the situation must be rewarding for the child. He must see it as worthwhile. The orange juice was the obvious reward in the first instance. In the second example the child was rewarded with a smile for looking at the speaker, and then praised for the castle she made. The children should not be told to 'look at me' only to be given a reprimand for inattention. This is clearly both unrewarding and a failure to understand the developmental stage of attention. This needs to be carefully explained and demonstrated to parents.

Constant training of this sort leads to the child gradually taking over the control of his own attention, so that he spontaneously gives his full attention to directions, provided that it has proved rewarding for him to do so during the learning stages.

(d) *Stage 4:* At the beginning of stage 4, the child's control of his attention focus may be rather slow, so that it is important he should be allowed time to stop what he is doing and look at the speaker, and then allowed time to transfer the directions to the task. A preliminary alerting signal may be needed such as calling the child's name, 'listen Johnny', or 'look at this', so that he has time to adjust his full attention before the directions are given. As he moves towards the stage of integration (level 5) he can assimilate the first part of the message while carrying on what he is doing, and he then looks at the speaker for completion of the directions. Once this control of attention focus is with the child, direct teaching is no longer necessary in order to achieve the subsequent stages. However, it is still very important to adjust communications to his level of attention control. Constantly overloading his attention at this stage, or failing to allow enough adjustment time, could cause a regression to earlier stages and habits of inattention. If anything is made too difficult for a child, with no hope of success, he will soon cease to try.

(e) *Stages 5 and 6:* These are the stages of integrated attention described in chapter 3. As far as teaching is concerned, the children can now respond to 'class' directions, and comply with simple instructions without having to interrupt a task. It is still important for teachers and parents to understand the limitations in terms of the sort of directions they are giving. If a child is doing up his shoelaces (a very difficult task for a 5 year old) he is unlikely to take in a complicated verbal message at the same time; but if he is drawing a picture, and the teacher says, 'put your pencils away, its play time', the message will be understood despite the fact that the child was visually occupied with a drawing. Again, no direct 'attention teaching' is needed at this stage, but rather an understanding of the limits and an adaptation of the communications.

Level 6 is the stage of well integrated and well sustained attention. This is the ultimate aim for this aspect of development in the developmental language programme. This stage is not achieved by all infant-school children, whether they are handicapped or not. Children who have attained this level of attention control are more than school ready in this area of development.

(2) *Performance abilities*

This includes visual perception, visuo-motor abilities and concept formation; areas of mainly non-linguistic intellectual development which have been described in chapter 3.

Visual perception and visuo-motor understanding lead to the building up of concepts, and it is the symbolization of these concepts which becomes language. Work on these areas must, therefore, go along with the more direct language work, even though there may not be specific handicaps in these aspects of learning.

(a) *Visual perception:* Visual perception is not a high level intellectual process in itself, but it becomes a way through to higher processing levels such as the formation and interrelation of concepts. It is with this progression in mind that the early work on visual perception is designed. Shape matching, such as form boards, and easy jigsaw puzzles, should lead on to more complex perceptual tasks such as finding two things the same out of a set of three. Real objects or very simple symbols are used at first. For example, a series consisting of two cups and a teapot. The child is not expected to tell, at this stage, why the cups and not the teapot are matched, but if the teacher brings in simple language it helps to move the task on towards the level of concepts, e.g. 'cup, cup, teapot'. This can lead to similar work with pictures. In this way the understanding moves on through gradual stages to more sophisticated perceptual differences such as line drawings of three carts, two with a dog in and one with Teddy in. At this stage a child would be expected to attempt some explanation of his choice of the two that are the same, even if this is only 'dog, dog, Teddy'. Visual perception at this level may become a training for reading readiness, as reading involves similar types of visual discrimination.

(b) *Visuo-motor abilities:* These are the sort of tasks in which the teacher builds a simple three-dimensional model, or a block design, and the child is required to copy it. This is rather more complex than visual perception in that it involves translating a visually perceived pattern into a pattern of motor movement in order to construct a similar one. If a child has difficulty with this type of task, the teacher will need to break it down into easier stages to find out which particular process is difficult for the child and help him with this. There may, for example, be a particular difficulty with colour, or with understanding position. When the area of difficulty has been isolated, the teacher needs to find ways of simplifying this aspect of the task so that it is within the child's understanding. In the early stages it is best to give the child the exact number of bricks for reproducing the model (e.g. block bridge), and to use only one colour. Three or four bricks are enough to start with, taking the child through the stages of towers, walls and bridges as set out on the record sheet. Sometimes it is difficult for a child to follow the construction of a model if the teacher is sitting opposite him. This has to be done from beside him so that he can, at first, copy the exact movements. A very simple verbal commentary may be introduced when the child is ready for this, as a help with the early stages of using language as a directive-integrative function. In addition to becoming the basis of simple concept formation, this sort of visuo-motor task can eventually become the foundation of paper and pencil work.

(c) *Constructional activities:* The children gradually move towards creating their own models without the need for an example to copy. This is a higher level, when they can translate their own inner ideas creatively in the form of spontaneous constructions with bricks or a more plastic material such as clay. Large sacks of bricks are useful in helping children to develop these constructive abilities. Left to themselves, they make towers or roads, but it is important for the teacher to help this on to more advanced stages, rather than just leaving the children to play. Suggestions such as putting a bridge over a road, or a house beside it, may help the child to create a more imaginative model. It also helps him to use language (adult's language at first) in planning and monitoring his activities.

(3) *Concept formation*

This involves the ability to move beyond the immediate percept towards abstractions such as size, shape and colour, understood as transferable attributes. This sort of conceptual thinking is the most 'central' of all intellectual processes, and becomes the pacemaker of all other aspects. There can be no meaningful symbol without a concept. This area of teaching is, therefore, very important at every age. The development of concepts has been described in chapter 3, and the teaching programme follows these stages.

(a) *One-to-one matching:* Experience has shown that colours are easier than shapes, so these are taught first, starting with a simple one-to-one match in which colour is the only variable, e.g. three cardboard circles of the same size, coloured red, yellow and blue, to be matched one-to-one to an exactly similar set. This can be followed by matching a set of coloured squares in the same way; then perhaps a set of coloured cups (must be all the same size and shape, varying only in colour). Then a set of three coloured cups may be matched to three coloured saucers; or three coloured spoons to three coloured plates. Later when the child can match colours using different objects, the property of colour has truly been abstracted as a concept, e.g. a set of three cups (yellow, red and blue) matched to a saucer, plate and spoon (red, yellow and blue). At this stage it is important to label the concepts using a word or sign, whichever the child can understand.

(b) *Classification:* At this stage, the abstraction, or generalized concept, can be understood as a guiding principle in sorting tasks, and precedes the percept. The first teaching stage is sorting objects into two categories only, according to either colour, shape or type. A box of beads of two different colours, for example, may be sorted into red and yellow; or a set of cutlery into forks and spoons. Three or more categories may be added as the child becomes ready for this.

Sorting into categories-by-use is more difficult. The concepts of use are more diffuse, and embrace a greater variety of objects. Children can be taught to achieve this level by sorting first according to familiar everyday use, such as things used for washing, and things used for eating. By this stage most children are able to manage sorting pictures, which are often easier to use and take up less space than objects. Some of the more intelligent children may be able to sort according to two categories at once, such as all the red things used for dressing; or all the green things used for eating. This stage is difficult for a child to understand without at least some understanding of language to identify the abstract concepts he is using.

The concepts of size and quantity are basic to all mathematical and numerical understanding. Teaching these concepts follows the same procedure as that described for colour and shape, starting with one-to-one matching, then two-category sorting, moving on to relative size and quantity using more than two categories. The record sheet gives the order in which these concepts are usually understood.

The understanding of 'same' is particularly difficult, but it is basic to so much of the concept work that it needs to be carefully and thoroughly taught. When the similarity can be directly perceived, as with shape and colour matching, this presents no special difficulty, but in the terms of quantity the understanding comes much later. Piaget (1974) has shown how perceptually dominated small children are in this sort of understanding. Something is more, or less, or the same only if it can be immediately perceived as such. These limitations need to be understood by the teacher who can only gradually take the child through to an understanding of the concepts which transcend the percepts. This becomes meaningful at first in terms of familiar material such as smarties or raisins. 'Who has more?', 'give everybody the same'.

Positional concepts are taught with language. Words may need to be accompanied by signs with some children. They are taught as true concepts, transferable to any material or situation, so that the child can, for example, understand that a cup is under the hat; that he is under the table; or later, that a picture shows a pair of shoes under the shelf. Real objects should be used first, and pictures introduced only when the positional concepts are really understood in three dimensions. The most usual order of difficulty is set out on the record sheet.

(4) *Symbolic understanding*

(a) *Representational play:* Much of the early teaching is concerned with helping the parents to play with their child. The need for representational play and its relationship to verbal language must be fully understood by the parents, and many of them need help in really coming down to child level to carry out this sort of play. Play sequences are carried out together with the therapist, parent and child all taking part in the session, so that parents get over their inhibitions and become able to enter into these play situations initiated by the therapist, at whatever level the child can understand. Play with large dolls can be carried out during the session, so that parents can use this same play in real-life situations at home. If the doll is also put to bed at the child's bedtime it helps him to understand that play can represent real situations, and that toys can represent, or symbolize real objects. If it is a home where there are no dolls (some parents will not give dolls to boys), then a Teddy or Panda can be used instead. Teddy can be fed at meal times, bathed at bath time (if it is washable!) and bedded at bedtime. This play, alongside real-life situations, helps in the early stages of understanding symbols. Later the play becomes meaningful in its own right, and scenes are enacted away from the real situation. Before this stage is reached, there may well be a long period in which the mother needs to initiate the play, and the child imitates her. Simple language is introduced alongside the play, e.g. 'Let's brush dolly's hair'. Even if the child is not ready to understand the words, this use of language in accompaniment to play creates an important communication situation between parent and child, and any response from the child, through play, can be very rewarding to the parents.

(c) *Small doll-play:* When the child really understands large doll-play and can play out simple sequences, he is ready for more symbolic material of small doll-play, material of doll's-house size. A few items of this sort played with on the table are better than an actual doll's house, which is too confined. The same sort of simple everyday sequences are acted out by the therapist with the child and parent, using these small toys when the child is ready for this. Language is increasingly introduced as an accompaniment to the actions with the toys, and can help to build up verbal comprehension. The parents can be shown how to initiate this sort of small doll-play so that sequences are meaningful to the child who gradually joins in and later initiates his own.

(c) *Pictures:* Parents often need help in understanding that pictures are not meaningful material until children are well able to understand three-dimensional symbols such as doll-play. Children may enjoy sitting on their mothers' knee looking at a picture book, at a much earlier age, and may even learn, through much repetition, to point to a particular picture in response to a particular word, but this does not necessarily mean that they understand that the picture represents a real object or situation. When pictures are introduced, this should be alongside the objects they represent at first. A picture of a cup is matched to the object cup, so that it is seen as truly representative rather than as a coloured pattern which, although attractive, may be without representational meaning. Matching objects to pictures is easiest with pictures cut out and stuck on cards. They should be clear coloured pictures, with only one object per card, such as those in the Ladybird Picture Book series. Parents may play a game in which the child finds the object about the room in response to the picture. For example, he goes to get an orange when shown the picture of an orange. This can be useful with children who are restless and active, and do not readily sit down to play.

In helping children to move from object-picture matching to toy-picture matching (symbol to symbol), it is helpful if the match is at first guided by clear perceptual similarities such as matching picture of a green car to a green toy car. This is to help the learning stage, but should move fairly quickly on to true symbol matching where these props are not needed. The aim is to get the child to match at the level of concepts rather than percepts, which means that each symbol must be translated into concept before the match can be made.

(d) *Gestures:* Gestures, like any other language form, move through stages which become increasingly symbolic. At first there are the near-direct communications such as pointing or holding out the arms for 'come'. This leads to mime, such as folding the hands on the cheek and shutting the eyes for 'sleep'. This is the stage of understanding that is particularly useful with pre-school children who have language handicaps. The more abstract hand signs such as the Paget Gorman sign system may be needed with a few children, but should be used selectively. At all levels gestures are used together with the spoken word, and never instead of this.

Although gestures are used freely by the teacher or therapist, in order to give the child every possible chance of understanding communications, the introduction of a systematic sign system is used very selectively, as not all the children need this. It can be useful as a way through for children who are afraid to attempt a vocal response. Once they have begun to communicate in this way, these children usually start to attempt vocal language, and this gradually takes over. Signs can also be useful for children who have word-finding difficulties. An alternative symbol seems to help them find the word. The rare child with a primary and persisting receptive aphasia may also need this form of communication. Most pre-school children need hand signs only as a prop in the learning stages and can dispense with them fairly quickly.

(e) *Written labels:* These may be introduced well before school age if the children are ready. Children aged 4+ years who have good verbal comprehension but a considerable expressive language problem, may be helped by the alternative medium of written labels. Because they have a difficulty with the spoken language it does not necessarily mean that the written language will also be difficult, so this alternative may be a help to some children.

(d) *Reading readiness:* It is important that children who have language handicaps should be given every chance to prevent a similar problem with reading, so 'reading readiness' activities are introduced to those children who are intellectually ready. This has already been mentioned under the heading of visual perception (p. 51). Work on sequencing can be helpful. Many language-handicapped children have difficulty with the sequence of sounds in words, or ordering words in sentences. Sequencing activities with objects and visual symbols (e.g. pictures) can sometimes help. Very early activities such as acting out the process of making and pouring out tea can move on through gradual stages to more complex activities such as putting pictures in the appropriate order for a story. This type of ordering can be useful as a foundation for reading, which is another form of ordering visual symbols.

(5) *Verbal comprehension*

In the early stages work on verbal comprehension is very much more important than expressive language. Young children with serious language handicaps need to have some soundly based understanding of language before really meaningful expressive language can be produced, and at each stage the understanding should precede the expression. Language cannot become an effective cognitive process if it is just 'talk'. Children vary as to how far the understanding needs to develop before language expression begins. The patterns of resolution in terms of this balance have been described in a previous publication (Reynell 1972). It is not always easy to get parents to understand the need for concentrating on receptive language, because a failure to 'talk' may be seen as the manifest handicap, but it is important to give them this understanding, so that they will concern themselves with verbal comprehension and reward progress in this aspect of development. A great deal of early work is concerned with getting the parents to monitor their own language with the child, so that it comes within the range of understanding. This means using short sentences with a clear message directly related to a concrete situation which is here and now. Parents need help in using appropriate sentence forms at each stage of development, adjusted to the child's level of understanding. This is combined with the teaching and use of his attention so that each communication may be as meaningful as possible. Parents are encouraged to use complete sentences, but with a number of 'operative' words carefully monitored, with the use of appropriate stresses. If, for example, the child can just manage to assimilate two named objects, appropriate sentences would be: 'put the cup on the table'; 'put the towel on the chair'; 'put your shoes on the doormat'. As always in the parent programme, this is built in to daily living situations so that communications become meaningful at home. When parents become aware of their role in this sort of teaching, they easily fall into the habit of adjusting their speech to the child, so that it does not inhibit natural communication, but rather enhances it.

Another aspect which needs plenty of demonstration to parents, is the need for immediate concrete reference if language is to be meaningful in the early stages. Transcending time and space with language cannot occur until a child has the ability to use verbal language as a thinking process. Constant questions such as 'where did we go the other day with Auntie?'; 'tell the teacher what we are going to do tomorrow?'; 'what did you do at school to-day?', these are well beyond the ability of a young language-handicapped child. He is more likely to be able to respond to 'who's that?'; 'what is she doing?', where the situation and related language are present in time and place.

Demonstration of these aspects of language learning is carried out during the session with parents and child, in situations related to daily living, using the sort of material available in that particular home. Parents can be shown, for example, that although a child can select a toy bus in response to naming, he cannot understand 'did you come here in a bus to-day?'

Parents and teachers need to be aware of the importance of rewarding success in verbal comprehension. It is easy enough to say 'good boy' when a child names something correctly, but the same need for reward applies when he carries out an appropriate action in response to a verbal request.

In a class situation, where teaching is more deliberate, suggestions for teaching different stages of verbal understanding, following the stage of understanding simple verbal labels, is as follows:

(a) *Relating two named objects:* This can be taught by using pairs of objects, changing only one of the pair at a time at first, e.g. 'put the spoon in the box'; 'put the fork in the box'; 'put the fork on the plate'. This gradually leads to the ability to relate any two named objects from a set of six or more. Then the child is ready to move on to relating nouns and verbs.

(b) *Relating nouns and verbs:* This is most easily taught by using small doll-play material, getting the child to set up play situations in response to verbal directions, or to identify situations set up by the teacher, e.g. 'show me the man sitting down'; 'where is the boy sleeping?' The present tense is used at first until the noun-verb concept is really understood. Pictures may be used instead of toys but they are often less attractive to children in the early stages. Picture material is more readily available, so once understanding has begun, and the child's interest can be held more easily, it may be more expedient to transfer to pictures. Small groups of children can be taught together in this sort of situation.

(c) *Relating nouns and adjectives and understanding long sentences:* These stages of understanding can also be taught with small toys, pictures or real objects, provided the children really understand the concepts being used. For example, it is not appropriate to give the direction 'show me the longest pencil' until the child understands the concept of relative length. This illustrates the need to understand all aspects of development and make the best use of every asset the child has while keeping the requests within his conceptual ability.

By the time the child can follow directions relating to three or more concepts, he is usually school ready in this aspect of development. He can now follow directions such as 'put the brown pencil in the drawer'; 'take the biggest ball out of the box'. He can also begin to understand language which extends beyond the here and now, using past and future tenses, e.g. 'This afternoon we are going to the park.'

(6) *Expressive language*

In the early stages very little direct teaching takes place in expressive language, until a sound basis of verbal comprehension is established. Parents are helped to understand the child's expressive language level so that their expectations may be realistic, and so they may reward at that level rather than continually demanding more. They need to focus on the more central aspects of language, in other words the content, in terms of attempts at words and phrases, rather than on sounds. At assessment some parents comment 'he doesn't say the ends of words', or 'he can't say his s's properly', when the child's actual language level is still at the stage of not more than a few meaningful words. They need to understand the developmental progression of expressive language, from situational jargon patterns, through words and phrases, short sentences, and finally the right coding of sounds in words. Any attempt at a word or phrase should be picked up, and reinforced by corrective feed-back, even if the sounds are so deviant that the attempt can only be recognized in context. For example, the child may say 'ere do-ee' which is reinforced with 'yes, there's dolly'. It is important that the feed-back is in fact what the child tried to say, otherwise this can be more confusing than helpful. Correction of the child's attempts at words and phrases should be avoided in the early stages, not only is this discouraging for the child, but it takes the sound production away from its related meaning at a stage of development when this relationship is precarious anyway. If his word for table is 'day', this should be accepted and rewarded, provided it is consistent and a true specific label as far as he is concerned.

When a child is ready to move on, this should be encouraged by helping him to expand his utterances. This can be done (i) by extended feed-back, but always within possible limits in terms of his level of ability; (ii) by giving him part of the extended sentence to complete; and (iii) by direct questions. Examples are:

(i) 'Dis bus goes'; 'Yes, this bus goes along the road.'
(ii) T, 'What is the boy doing? He is. . . .'
(iii) T, 'Tell me what is happening.'

As with verbal comprehension, the focus is on an on-going activity with concrete material, or play with toys. This makes the language immediately meaningful and takes the focus off the very inhibiting 'question-answer' situation. There are plenty of opportunities in daily living to help children form sentences in this way as the following exemplifies:

Mother drops a potato on the floor.
M: 'Oh, what happened?'
Child: 'Tato falled.'
M: 'Yes the potato fell on the floor'.

Careful guidance is needed by the speech therapist or teacher to ensure that the sort of language expansion used is appropriate for the child's level of ability. He should be gently taken on to the next developmental stage, but not jumped several stages ahead.

Some children, such as those with a word-finding difficulty, may be helped by using a sign as an intermediary, but this can be dropped as soon as the word is readily available to the child.

The early developmental stages for expressive language are very similar to those for verbal comprehension, but each stage develops a little later.

(7) *Articulation:* It is not advisable to focus the child's attention on correction of articulation in the early stages of language development, although corrective feed-back on the part of the adult is appropriate. In order for the child to make this correction he needs to be mature enough to divorce the sounds from the content without destroying the content. This level of maturity is unusual at the early stages considered in this developmental programme. That is the reason why this aspect of language production is not given too much emphasis in the programme.

When children have reached the stage where focus on articulation becomes appropriate, they should have reached the level where language has already become a useful cognitive process. By this time they are beginning to move beyond the need of some of the developmental areas of this language programme and more direct 'speech' work can take over. Many children who have been through the developmental language programme do need this final aspect of language help on entering school. It is often more appropriate for this to be given by the speech therapist on a weekly or intensive basis.

(8) *Intellectual use of language*

The use of language as a directive-integrative function, helping to plan and monitor play and activities, and finally becoming an important internalized intellectual process, is the ultimate aim of the developmental language programme. It is important that this aim should be considered all the time, at all stages, and that the child be encouraged and helped in the use of language in this way at every stage. The stages in the development of this function of language have been described in chapter 3.

(a) *Stage 1: Pre-integration:* Parents need a great deal of help in understanding that their well-intentioned verbal directions to their child may not help him, because he cannot yet manage the integration of verbal directions with his activities. Verbal bombardment can be very disturbing to a child who needs all his attention for whatever he is doing. This was illustrated by a retarded four year old (see p. 34) who was playing well with the symbolic toys until her father started to bombard her with verbal directions. She had to stop the play and put her hands over her ears to cope with the distress he was causing her. At this early stage a very simple verbal accompaniment is all that is appropriate; taking the form of an intermittent commentary coincidental with the actions, e.g. 'Dolly's having a bath'; 'cup of tea for Dolly'. The commentary should not be more than the child can tolerate, of course, and should be shortened or stopped altogether at the first sign that it is interfering with the child's play or activity. Familiar situational phrases are enough at first. The speech therapist can guide the parents on how much their child is ready to take at each stage, to help him on the next stage, when adult verbal guidance can be an asset.

(b) *Stage 2: Adult verbal guidance helps:* When the child has reached the stage at which the adult's verbal commentary can move on to simple suggestions in anticipation of immediate actions, then he is ready for work at stage 2. At this stage the verbal guidance is not just a simple accompaniment to play, but helps to plan and guide the activities, e.g. 'Let's put dolly in the bath', 'shall we give her a cup of tea?' At first the verbal guidance is very simple and only precedes an action which is likely to happen anyway, but gradually it can take the form of true suggestions to modify and help the activity or play, e.g. 'Build another road', 'put a brick on top'. This is obviously closely bound up with the child's verbal comprehension level and this must be considered in the type of directions given. Also his understanding of concepts and symbols may set certain limits which need to be understood.

(c) *Stage 3:* When he can really use adult verbal guidance, integrating this with his play and activities in a way which helps the activities to achieve a higher level, the child is ready to take on this role for himself. He can be helped to do this by gentle prompting during his play, first of all in accompaniment and later in planning his activities, e.g. 'the car is going under the bridge ... what is the car doing?' and later, 'where will the car go?' Language-handicapped children may need to prolong this stage of externalizing their own verbal guidance beyond the usual age. It is important that teachers at the receiving Infant Schools should understand this, and not tell the child to 'be quiet and get on with your work'. Instead he could be told 'talk very quietly, James'. This will help him gradually to internalize his own verbal guidance so that it becomes a whisper, and finally an internalized thinking process, when he reaches stage 4.

The role of the speech therapist in the classroom

It is advisable for a qualified teacher to have charge of a language class, as this involves professional skills such as group management and certain teaching techniques for which speech therapists are not trained. On the other hand speech therapists can contribute other professional skills that the teachers do not have. The speech therapist's contribution to a language class should be such that her professional skills and time are used to the best advantage. A full time speech therapist is not essential and few speech therapists can spare this amount of time to such a small number of children, but there should be enough allowance of time to cover the following:

(i) Carrying out language assessments on or before admission and at annual review. Also, on-going assessment of specific aspects of language in individual cases.

(ii) Discussions with the teacher on programme planning, and advice on specific aspects of language help needed for individual children.

(iii) Individual work with children who are ready for this. This is often appropriate as children resolve the more central aspects of their difficulties and need a more direct focus on sentence construction, or in coding the right sounds in words.

(iv) Work on a modified parent programme alongside the class work is highly desirable, if there is enough speech therapy time available, and would enable the children to have the maximum amount of on-going help.

There can be no hard and fast rules about 'who does what', as this must depend on the particular situation and the availability of specialist help. The roles should be carefully thought out in each case when setting up a language class, so that professional time is used to the best advantage. Language classes are expensive in professional time, as compared to the parent programme, so it is particularly important to plan allocation of professional time very carefully.

The suggestions made in this chapter are applicable to parents working with children at home under the guidance of the speech therapist and to children in special classes or special schools. The case illustrations in the following chapter will bring the suggestions alive in a more specific way, with examples of children in the parent programme and in the class programme.

Chapter 6 Case illustrations

The following three children were referred to an assessment centre and after assessment were placed either in the parent clinic or class programme:

Philip in the parent clinic programme at 2 years 5 months
Sally in the parent clinic programme at 3 years and then transferred to the class programme at 4 years 2 months
Tom in the class programme at 3 years 10 months.

Philip

Philip was referred to the Centre by his family doctor at the age of two years and five months, because of speech and language delay.

Philip's parents felt that his general development had been within normal limits but they did consider he had been a rather quiet baby, who did not babble until after he was one year old. It was only in the last two or three months prior to referral, that he had responded to the verbal cue rather than a gesture for 'bye bye' and had started using a few labels. The parents also reported that he had become progressively more difficult to manage, that he was easily frustrated and often very provocative in his behaviour. At the time of referral he was their only child. The parents had both had further education leading to professional qualification. The mother had a history of depressive illness.

Assessment

Philip presented as a little boy of normal appearance but with some immaturity in locomotor and manipulative skills, unaccompanied by any classic neurological deficit.

Hearing was normal.
The psychological assessment showed his non-verbal abilities to be well up to his chronological age (2.5 years).
Attention control was at level 2.

Symbolic understanding was at a level where he recognized but did not use large doll material—apparently having little idea of play. This level was below 2 years.

Verbal comprehension: Philip recognized labels but was only just moving to a level where he could assimilate a simple command (e.g. put the *spoon* in the *cup*). This was at a 1 year 10 months level on the Reynell Scales.

Expressive language: He had only six recognizable words, although he made some attempts to name objects. On the Reynell Scales he rated at 1 year 5 months.

Clinic programme

On the first visit in the clinic programme, Philip came with both parents and Father mainly handled the child, although both parents appeared very willing to cooperate. On most subsequent visits only Mother attended and he was always calmer when Father was not in attendance.

Throughout the work in the clinic, it was emphasized that pre-language and language should relate to daily environmental activities.

Attention control work: The need to gain Philip's full attention was demonstrated. Also, the need to concentrate on single channel situations; in other words, the need to stop any activity and get Philip's full attention to an auditory stimulus (e.g. putting rings on a holder in response to a speech sound). When Philip was able to do this sort of activity quite easily, we were able to demonstrate how he could be encouraged to control his own activities (e.g. when carrying out a command—to stop activity and look at the speaker).

Symbolic understanding: At first it was necessary to demonstrate the use of large doll material in play. This was discussed with Mother and it was found he had little of this sort of toy material but Mother was very willing to develop this form of play. We were then able to demonstrate the use of small doll material and then object picture matching. Mother was able to join in these activities, although it was apparent that this had not previously been carried out at home. She was rewarded by Philip's response to her interaction in this play situation. Philip developed quickly through the various developmental levels of symbolic understanding.

Verbal comprehension: It was necessary to demonstrate Philip's limited level of language comprehension (labelling ability was only just developing) and therefore the need to restrict the amount of 'input'. Mother had felt that the more information she 'fed in' the more helpful to Philip. She recognized his difficulty to cope but found some difficulty herself in restricting her own language and needed constant reminders and encouragement to reduce the complexity of her verbal messages. After the first two or three sessions she had begun to do this. It was also necessary to demonstrate the need for language at first to be always related to the 'here and now' situation.

Verbal comprehension work was started with much labelling of objects which were meaningful to Philip. Later, object linking and then noun and verb phrases were demonstrated. Always using these as and when occasion arose in play or environmental situations (e.g. 'put the *man* on the *chair*', then later 'show me the *man* who is *sleeping*'; still later 'show me the *man* who is driving the *car*', etc.).

Expressive language: This aspect of language was not emphasized at first in the programme. The importance of the more fundamental aspects of language was stressed, and explained to his Mother. As his verbal comprehension improved, he was then encouraged to attempt labelling objects; and to link two labels; and later to link label and activity words together. This was demonstrated to Mother in a play situation, asking Philip to give her certain objects and then later setting up simple scenes, e.g. small doll in a bed and asking Philip to tell her about it, accepting at first phrases such as 'girl ... bed' and feeding back the correct phrase 'yes, the girl is in the bed'; later expecting 'girl sleep' or 'girl sleeping' and using the corrective feedback 'yes, the girl is sleeping'. At a later stage this could be expanded to 'yes, the *girl* is *sleeping* in bed', etc.

Articulation was at first immature but parents were advised not to be concerned about this only to use corrective feedback rather than attempt to get Philip to correct this.

Progress

Philip was once more re-assessed at the age of five years. He was now attending normal infant school.

He still presented as a lively child but his energy and drive were now directed towards achievement.

Attention control: fully mature for a school-age child (level 6).

Verbal comprehension: now well above his chronological age. On Reynell Scale 6.3 years.

Expressive language: now consistent with his age (level 5.4 years), although he still showed immaturities in articulation which it was felt should now resolve spontaneously. Philip was now using language well in his own thinking and reading at an appropriate age level.

Sally

Sally was referred for assessment at the age of 2 years 10 months, with a history of general delay in development, with a specific 'speech delay'. At the time of referral she was the only child of professional parents.

Assessment

At 3 years, Sally was seen as a solid, chubby child, clumsy in movement, very cautious and clinging. She was very quiet and slow to respond to sound. She tended to become absorbed in handling objects but this was inclined to be a repetitive and a non-creative play situation. Occasionally Sally would demonstrate odd outbursts of energy.

Paediatric assessment did not reveal any clear cause for her developmental delay, and her hearing was found to be within normal limits.

Psychological assessment showed Sally's non-verbal performance abilities to be approximately a year below her chronological age.

Attention control was at a developmental level where she was easily distracted by any stimulus (level 1).

Symbolic understanding was at a level where she recognized large doll-play material, but she did not play with it (approximately 18 months).

Verbal comprehension: Sally recognized some verbal labels when produced by Mother in a familiar situation, but could not manage these when given by another adult. On the Reynell Verbal Comprehension Scale she rated at 1 year 7 months.

Expressive language: Sally produced a few vocalizations in play but none of them were real verbal labels. On the Reynell Expressive Language scale she scored at 9 months.

Use of language: On referral, Sally was at the stage where adult language interfered with her activities and she was in no way able to make use of it (stage 1).

Parent clinic programme

Sally attended regularly with her mother. Father could attend only very occasionally. Mother appeared very cooperative and keen to gain insight and understanding of the principles involved in helping Sally. It was understood that Father was also interested and that Mother passed on the advice given at each session.

Symbolic understanding: It was necessary to spend much time in the first few sessions helping Mother to play with Sally, recreating familiar home routines with a large doll, e.g. feeding the dolly, dressing it, putting it to bed, etc. It was also necessary to help Mother monitor the quality of her own language with Sally. She had not previously talked to her very much and when she did, it was often too linguistically sophisticated and not sufficiently related to the 'here and now' situation. We demonstrated how simple language could accompany play sequences and encouraged Mother to participate in this, so that we could at first monitor her language input to Sally.

Mother was keen to take Sally to a play group once or twice a week and we agreed that this might be helpful for Mother to see play activities with other children, and adult involvement in that situation. We explained that Sally would, however, learn more easily from adults than from other children.

As large doll-play improved, we gradually introduced smaller toy objects—carrying out simple everyday experiences with these toys, e.g. mother dolly and toy cooker/dolly in toy bath/daddy dolly sitting on toy chair, etc. Later, as play developed, we began object/object matching and object/toy matching and towards the end of the time in the clinic programme, we had just begun to introduce picture/object matching but this was still very precarious and only at a perceptive level, at the time Sally entered the language class programme.

Attention control: This was, perhaps, one of Sally's greatest learning handicaps at first, and it was very important to help Mother to gain Sally's attention and gradually to teach her to control her own attention, so that she could benefit from a learning situation. We devised games to encourage this (using any noise-making toys we had) making a noise to which Sally would then respond by listening and then immediately rewarding her for doing so. At first such games were only part of the attention training but they were helpful. It gave Mother something specific to do, and as Sally improved, it was also rewarding. It was necessary, however, for Mother to learn to gain Sally's full attention in any task she was undertaking and we encouraged her to get full facial attention whenever she was directly speaking to her.

She moved slowly to attention level 2 and here it was necessary for Mother to understand Sally's difficulty in shifting attention. She needed at first to accept Sally's own choice of task or toy material, only gently intervening and extending the play, e.g. Sally would choose to play with dolly and would play out the sequence of taking her clothes off and washing her. We would then suggest we dry dolly with the towel and put her to bed. This at first would be met by irritated squeals and a return to the task of washing dolly. Gradually we encouraged the next step, until she learnt that 'drying dolly' and putting her to bed was all part of the task she had chosen and carried out the sequence herself.

Verbal comprehension: When we first saw Sally in the clinic, she was not able to select objects by any verbal label. With Mother she was able to do so for a few objects with very clear situational clues, e.g. at meal time Mother would ask Sally to give her her mug—and this Sally could do. We encouraged Mother to increase this form of recognition, asking for familiar objects in varied situations, e.g meal times, bath times, dressing, undressing, and gradually in the play situations. After the first two visits, Sally was able to do this for us with some degree of consistency and we suggested it was time to link two familiar objects by name, e.g put your *shoe* on the *chair*, put *dolly* in the *bed*, etc. Mother understood that this was not just an exercise carried out once a day, but an on-going situation which she could encourage as she and Sally went around the home together, while she was doing the housework and cooking and also in activities when she was more directly involved with her, at bedtime, bath time and in play, etc.

Expressive language: As can be seen from the initial assessment, she had no recognizable words and this was naturally the greatest area of concern for the parents. We needed to emphasize how an initial approach to this problem must first be to improve attention control and the understanding of symbols and the receptive aspects of language. As these aspects made some headway, so Sally's vocalizations increased both in terms of quantity and variety. We suggested that Mother constantly reinforce these vocalizations, feeding back the appropriate word or phrase.

Class programme

At 4.2 years we felt Sally was ready for more intensive teaching and that she was mature enough to be separated from Mother. At first she found this very difficult, hiding behind Mother's back and squeaking whenever an adult approached her. At first she came with Mother and escort on the 'school' bus. She had already met the class staff, so we were not entirely unfamiliar. After a week she allowed the teacher to work alongside Mother, but it was another week before she would allow Mother to leave the classroom. Mother would then wait in the reception area and Sally would be taken out to see her as often as she requested during the session. The next stage of separation was when Mother came with her but then left, and Sally would go home with the escort. By the middle of the third week, Sally was able to come to the class unaccompanied by Mother.

Attention control: Sally had achieved level 2 in the clinic situation and even occasionally level 3. On entry to the class, she regressed to level 1 and so specific training in control was again used, taking her alone in a quiet corner until she could tolerate the group situation. Within about a month, Sally was back at level 2 and moving steadily towards level 3. She needed constant help, however, and directions such as 'Stop, Sally—look at me' giving her time to assimilate the instruction and rewarding her whenever this was achieved. By the time she left the class, she was achieving level 4 in attention control, now able to control this without constant help from the adult. She was still not able to integrate both verbal and visual stimuli while carrying out a task.

Non-verbal abilities: On entry to the class, her performance ability was at 2.10 year level on the Griffiths scale. She could do simple insert boards and build a tower. At first, the teaching aim was to slow down Sally's attempts at the task, helping her to gain better hand control. She was inclined to rush at the task, clumsily dropping and knocking things over, saying all the while 'I ca—I ca' (I can). In the early stages of teaching the building of models, she was given a model and then helped step by step to reproduce this. We considered learning was really consolidated when she could reproduce these models, using different materials, e.g. building a bridge with bricks, and then perhaps with two yoghurt cartons and a piece of paper.

Visual perceptual abilities: She was able to match simple shapes but needed help to develop this task. At first she was given two halves of an identical complete shape—matching these to a model—then the model was removed; she was given one half of the shape and had to select the appropriate half to complete the task. Progress accelerated in this area and before leaving the class she had reached a 4 year level.

Symbolic understanding: As Sally had reached the stage of understanding large clear pictures, these formed the basis of material for teaching in other areas together with the use of small toys.

Concept formation: On entry to the class, she was functioning mainly at a perceptual level, without the ability to make abstractions or generalizations. Teaching began with one-to-one matching of colours, shapes and objects, bringing names in to help to form the concepts, e.g. a square was called 'a square like a window', 'a triangle like a roof', etc. Sally was not at first expected to use the names herself. It was not necessary for each concept to be consolidated before introducing another one, i.e. shapes before colours, etc. and this helped to prevent her from becoming bored.

We then taught classification in sorting colours, shapes and objects. Coloured beads and bricks were used, making sure the colour shades were the same. In the early stages, shapes were the same size, colour and texture, but gradually variations were introduced.

Relative sizes were taught later, starting with big and small (little) using cues to help, such as putting all the big bricks in a big box, the small ones in a small box. Paget Gorman signs were also used to reinforce the use of a 'big' or 'little' voice. Learning was consolidated when she had learnt to do this task with pictures. When she had learnt a number of concepts, she was taught how to sort objects into categories by use and by the time she left the class, she could do this with pictures.

Verbal comprehension: On entry to the class, she was linking two named objects, but these needed to be consolidated and extended before moving on to relating nouns and verbs. We taught one verb at a time and used the present tense. Scenes were set up with small toy material, e.g. boy sitting, girl sitting, lady sitting, and Sally was asked to 'show me the girl sitting', etc. Later, scenes were set up with more choices and then action pictures were used. Noun/adjective links followed quite quickly, as concepts like colour, shape and size were understood.

Expressive language: On entry to the class, she was using a number of recognizable words and some situational phrases, and the work at first was aimed mainly at extending her naming vocabulary and reinforced by corrective feedback. The work in the class was also backed up by specific individual work with the speech therapists. As her vocabulary increased, it was evident that she had difficulty in finding words and she needed additional clues to help her, such as gesture and the picture of the object. In addition to the 'central' language problem, the tone of her voice indicated some structural difficulties and she was referred for investigation of this. No operative procedure was considered appropriate at this stage, although it was probable that there might be some disproportion of the palate in relation to the nasopharynx.

Use of language: She entered the class at the stage where adult language was proving helpful but she did not initiate language herself. She began to use language gradually, but only to gain the adult's attention, not to give or ask for information. With the other children she was cooperative in play but at first silent, and then cautiously she volunteered comments until finally, she was confident in this despite her obvious articulatory problem.

Progress

When Sally was 5 years 5 months, she had been in the class 15 months and it was decided she should enter school. The parents chose a Montessori School where she could continue in structured learning situations. For the first term she attended half-days only, continuing to attend for half-days in the language class. This enabled her to adjust to the new situation and we were able to build up a good liaison with the school.

On reassessment at 5 years 10 months, she had made steady progress in performance, now 4 years 10 months, and had made accelerated progress in both language areas.

Verbal comprehension: 3 years 10 months.

Expressive language: 2 years 10 months.

There was still a considerable gap between her verbal and non-verbal abilities, but this was seen to be gradually growing less as her language improved. There was an improvement in her attention control and in her social adjustment, and she was reported to have settled quickly and happily in school. We arranged for her to have continuing speech therapy.

Tom

Tom was referred to the Centre at three years and six months. He was referred by his family doctor because of developmental delay and behaviour difficulties.

His pre and peri-natal histories were essentially normal. He presented as a child with some degree of generalized retardation but with a superimposed communication handicap which was extensive and severe. There were behaviour difficulties secondary to his communication handicap, which made him difficult to manage at home. He had had ear infections in the past, but these had cleared up by the time of referral and were not thought to be a significant contributory factor to his present communication handicap.

Tom was the second child of a social class IV family. His mother was reported to be a late talker and had speech therapy as a child.

Assessment

Tom was physically big for his age, which made his intellectual and language retardation even more obvious. He was a very active child and when first seen in the reception area, he rushed around jumping on and off the large toys, pulling other children off any equipment he wanted and not appearing to relate to other children in any way. He tipped toys out from the box but did not play constructively with the material in this situation.

Psychological assessment showed his performance abilities were at a two years and four months level. In symbolic understanding he demonstrated some recognition of small toys but no imaginative play or classification. He was able to match toys and pictures and was considered to be at a two year level.

Attention control was at level 1.

Verbal comprehension: On the Reynell scales this was at a twelve months level. He was not able to select objects in response to naming but was able to follow some situational phrases.

Expressive language: He was at a one year and five months level. He was able to name some objects but only in free play. He was using a few jargon patterns but no recognizable word combinations.

Class programme

Tom was admitted to the language class at three years and ten months and remained in the class for fifteen months. He presented many problems besides his intellectual and language retardation. He was aggressive, destructive and non-compliant and he appeared to have no idea of self-preservation.

On admission he was still wearing nappies and incontinent.

For the first two weeks his mother attended with him to help him to settle. He appeared to ignore her and it was necessary to reassure her that this was only because of his interest in the new toys, etc. After Tom was settled in the class, his mother was invited at regular intervals to watch the teaching sessions and to discuss ways in which she could help. As his behaviour improved in class, he was easier to handle at home.

Initially, the foremost problem was his incontinence. He enjoyed social reinforcement, e.g. a hug or a kiss, and although this was good for the learning situation, it was difficult to cuddle him. Mother was asked to take him out of nappies and put him into trainer pants. She was at first reluctant but when it was indicated that we would undertake the toilet training, agreed to do so. Tom responded well to training and by the end of the first term was clean and dry in the class. He was taught a word for toilet and started to take himself there. He was rewarded with raisins and hugs during this training period. Getting him dry at home took longer, particularly at night, but Mother was helped with a programme of training and gradually this was achieved.

Tom's aggression and destructiveness caused distress to the other children. He seemed perplexed by their tears when he upset them, having little idea of cause and effect. We first tried a firm 'No Tom' holding his hands still when he went to grab another child's toy but this was not effective. We then tried 'time-out', removing him from the classroom for a few minutes and this was more successful, and as his language skills improved, we were able to control his behaviour by our own language.

Attention control: Work was at first carried out in a separate quiet room (not the one used for 'time-out'). He was taught to carry out a simple task on a given signal. This signal had to be the dominant stimulus and at first we used loud noise-makers—a variety were needed to hold his interest and he needed to have played with them for a few minutes before turning it into a listening activity. Later we were able to introduce quieter speech sounds and signal words. By that time he was able to carry out such tasks in a corner of the classroom. By the end of the first term he was just able to tolerate this task for five minutes. Slowly he moved on to level 2 and stayed at this level for a long time, so it was difficult to establish a very satisfactory teaching situation. At first he 'cut out' whenever language was introduced into the task and we had to play alongside him for a long time with his own choice of activity, only gradually being able to intervene and thus move him to level 3. When Tom left the class at 5 years 1 month, he had reached level 4 but this was still very immature for school entrance.

Performance: On all tasks Tom had to be presented with ones that provided a good possibility of success; otherwise he did not persevere. In visual perceptual tasks at first he could only match a circle to a circle and a square to a square. Gradually we introduced more shapes and he learned to match complex shapes to insets. Later, language was introduced so that he was required to 'tell' about the 'sameness' or difference. This was reinforced by use of Paget Gorman signs. In visuo-motor tasks, Tom could at first only build a tower or a wall if he copied it, but later he was able to have the model taken away and do this from memory. He finally achieved a level consistent with his chronological age in performance tasks.

Symbolic understanding: At first, all play sequences had to be achieved with adult modelling and later with adult verbal guidance. Tom in fact soon developed good imaginative role play and this served as an excellent base for language work.

Concept formation: It was necessary to work gradually from simple perceptual matching, using material such as bricks and beads, to the stage at which he was able to understand abstractions such as size and shape. This came with his ability to sort into categories. He needed many examples before any new concept was consolidated. At first we used concrete materials to teach new concepts and then two-dimensional material such as coloured pictures.

A good example of Tom's gradual development in moving from a simple colour-sorting task into a size-ordering task occurred when he was sorting a box of beads of various colours into three trays of different colours and different shapes. He was happily sorting into colours when suddenly he said, 'no no dis (this) big one, dis miggle (middle) one and dis likkle one.' He then put all the beads back into the box and began again, correctly carrying out a size-ordering task.

Verbal comprehension: It was difficult to gain Tom's attention to speech and it was a whole term before he was really interested in verbal labels. When this was achieved, it was then an equally slow teaching situation before Tom could cope with the next stage of relating two named objects. His attention had always to be set before each task and controlled by adult intervention: 'Stop, Tom—look at me—listen', etc. When Tom left the class he was, however, able to select objects in response to a description of their use and as concepts developed he was beginning to understand noun-adjective links, e.g. 'Put the *blue brick* in the *lorry*'. He was not, however, able to cope with 'Put the *little dog* on the *red chair*'.

Expressive language: This was not treated as a separate area of work but was linked always with verbal comprehension activities and thus worked on at the same level. For example, in asking Tom to 'put the dolly in the bath' this could lead to such questions as 'who is in the bath' and 'where is the dolly'. As this aspect of his language development was at first ahead of his comprehension, we did not emphasize the need to increase this to begin with, but rewarded Tom whenever he initiated a label or phrase. He had begun to be able to give short incomplete sentences when he left the class. Use of language as a directive-integrative function was at first not possible for Tom. At first it was necessary for us as adults to use verbal directions for our own guidance in a parallel play situation—gradually Tom also made use of this and by the time he left the class, he was beginning to use his own externalized verbal directions.

Progress

At five years one month (15 months after he entered our language class programme) he started in Infant School for half-days, continuing the other half of each day in our class for one term. Careful liaison was carried out with the school. His teacher visited the Centre and full reports were sent to the school. Local speech therapy was arranged on a weekly basis. On a follow-up visit to the school, Tom seemed at first a little confused in a somewhat unstructured classroom setting with a high noise level, although his behaviour was now much more cooperative and ready for a learning situation. However, on reassessment it was reassuring that he had maintained the progress made in the language class.

The results of this reassessment at five years and six months were as follows:

Concept formation: he was now able to extend his thinking beyond the immediately perceptual.

Attention control: was now at level 3 but this was still precarious at times. It was still at a pre-school level and therefore difficult for him in the classroom.

Verbal comprehension: was continuing to make good progress but he still got confused with longer sentences. He was functioning at a level of three years and nine months. He was now using language to express his ideas but generally talking in short incomplete sentences.

Chapter 7 Recording progress

In the foregoing chapters the theoretical basis and aims of the developmental language programme have been set out and the practical applications described. It is hoped that these chapters will enable many people working in different circumstances to help the language development of young children who may be in need of this. In itself, however, this is not enough unless it can really be shown that the aims are achieved, at least in part, for each child. For this purpose regular and careful record keeping is essential. It is not enough just to see 'progress', as some progress at a steady rate is likely to occur whether or not there is intervention. The aim of the developmental programme is to accelerate language development so that there is some catching up towards the level of the child's non-verbal abilities, which in turn may enhance total intellectual development.

The specific aims of the programme are to consolidate the child's present level in all the areas shown in Figure 2, and help him on to the next developmental stage. A clear understanding of the developmental stages is important so that the help given can really be used by the child. If teaching is at too high a level, several stages in advance, this will not reach the child. Similarly, if it is at too low a level it is not using the time to the best advantage in helping him to advance.

In order to help those who are carrying out the programme to keep all the stages of development in mind, and to remember where each child is, this has been set out on record sheets, as shown in the Appendix. These sheets also serve as individual records of progress.

Use of individual record sheets

Booklets can be made up for each child from the charts shown in the Appendix so that each page gives a record of progress in one area of development, such as attention control, concept formation, etc. At the time of assessment the child's level is established, and forms the first entry in the booklet on each page. Thus, if his attention control level is assessed as stable at level 2, ready to move on to level 3, the teacher or speech therapist can immediately see where to start helping the child. A three-point rating scale has been found useful for recording progress, so that at each stage of development the child's achievements can be rated as:

(i)　level achieved occasionally (blue dot);
(ii)　level achieved most of the time but still fluctuating (green dot);
(iii)　level stable and consolidated (red dot). When a particular level is consolidated, the child is ready to move on to the next developmental stage.

The developmental stages given in the record sheets cover the important stages up to school readiness and are therefore realistic in terms of the aims for pre-school children or older retarded children still intellectually at a pre-school level.

It is recommended that a record is made for each child at four to six-weekly intervals. This allows some time for progress to have been made, and yet is a short enough gap to make sure that the teaching is achieving its aims, without the necessity of waiting for an annual review.

In the Wolfson Centre study with pre-school children, these records proved to be not only an essential guide and record of progress, but were also very reliable in predicting school placement and early school success. Follow-up studies will be published when these data are complete. The indications are that this sort of progress record could have an additional importance in this respect for children in Observation and Assessment units.

To summarize: By using the record forms, the programme director can see at any time

(i) what level of work is appropriate for each child in each area of development,
(ii) what are the immediate aims in terms of learning stages,
(iii) how fast the child is progressing and in which areas,
(iv) whether an adequate balance is being maintained between one developmental area and another,
(v) how near the child is to school readiness in each area of development.

Progress rating

In using the developmental programme and recording progress it is important to understand the difference between a 'skill' and a true intellectual 'process'. A skill may be achieved by teaching always on the same material and in the same way, so that a specific skill such as a jigsaw puzzle may be achieved at a spuriously high level. If this is not fully understood by the teacher or speech therapist, a stage of development may be wrongly recorded as 'stable' when it only applies to the particular set of circumstances in which it was taught. This may lead to apparent regression during school holidays, and a failure to achieve the same level at different times and under different conditions. Teaching needs to be widely based so that it is, in the example given above, a true understanding of perceptual shape matching as an intellectual 'process', and not achievement on one particular puzzle which is taught and recorded. If the ability is achieved as a 'process' and not merely as a specific 'skill', it should be transferable to any material or situation which demands the same developmental stage in terms of understanding. In understanding verbal labels, for example, a child must be able to select named objects wherever they are, and in response to whoever asks for them. Likewise, in understanding the construction of simple 'bridges', the child must be able to do this with any set of bricks, boxes or other suitable material, of reasonable size, and be able to do this without help. Indeed it is an essential feature of the parent guidance programme that parents should understand what 'processes' are being demanded of a child in different circumstances and at different times during daily living.

The rating of progress, described above, must therefore be concerned only with the central 'process' and not with a particular skill which is situation bound.

Validation

Anyone who publishes a teaching programme has an obvious duty first of all to make sure, as far as possible, that the programme is 'valid' in that it does what it purports to do, when used by suitably qualified professional people. Early validation studies on the developmental language programme have already been published (Cooper *et al.* 1974), so will only be mentioned briefly here. Further studies have amply confirmed these findings and will be published when the data are complete.

Assessment of progress for individual children, each child acting as his own control, shows whether the aims have been achieved in terms of (a) progress in the different areas of development, and (b) measurable rate of progress over the year using standardized tests for which the norms are also equivalent to 'controls'. Assessment of the programme itself was attempted by comparing the rate of progress of the groups of children in the developmental language programme with that of groups of children of similar age and handicap who were (a) having no help and (b) were having weekly speech therapy locally. The findings indicated that for individual children the aims were achieved in terms of (a) progress towards school readiness in the different areas of development, and (b) acceleration of language development as assessed at annual review using standardized tests. These aims were achieved in well over 80 per cent of the Wolfson Centre sample. Group comparisons showed that children in the developmental language programmes made better progress than children in either control group.

On the basis of these findings the suggestions made in this volume can be put forward with some degree of confidence as a way of helping children to overcome early language handicaps.

Field trials

Validation studies with the Wolfson Centre sample have demonstrated the value of the developmental programme in helping children attending the language classes and those in the parent programme. However, there is still a need to know whether the programme is equally effective if carried out by other people in different types of setting, and with different samples of children. For these further studies, which are still on-going, we are indebted to the teachers and speech therapists who have agreed to use the programme under our direction, and allow us to carry out assessments of the children at the beginning and end of the year. These studies include classes in ESN(M) and ESN(S) schools, an assessment unit, and pre-school groups for language-handicapped children, for the class field trials. They also include children under the age of five, with a wide range of language handicaps, having help in the parent programme with speech therapists in different parts of the country. The reassessments so far carried out have been encouraging, suggesting that the validity may be maintained under these different conditions, but these field trials are still incomplete, and further details will be published later.

Appendix 1 Film

'Helping language development' version B

This 20 minute film is available for hire from the NFER Publishing Company Ltd. It illustrates the language intervention programme described in this handbook. It is a 16 mm sound film in colour.

The first part of the film shows three children having help in the 'parent' programme, and the second part shows the language class.

In order to achieve the conditions necessary for filming, and to show as many examples of the work as possible, the situations shown are necessarily more confined in time and space than they are in the actual situations, and this creates a somewhat false impression. For example, the language clinic sessions are not usually conducted entirely sitting at a table, but with the child free to move about the room; and the class situations are not quite so intense as they appear on film.

Despite these limitations the film should be helpful to those who wish to put into practice the ideas described in this handbook.

Appendix 2   Individual schedules

NAME:

D.O.B.:   DATE:

ATTENTION CONTROL												
1. CAN PAY FLEETING ATTENTION THOUGH HIGHLY DISTRACTIBLE												
2. RIGID ATTENTION TO OWN CHOICE OF ACTIVITY												
3. SINGLE CHANNEL ATTENTION: CAN ATTEND TO ADULT'S CHOICE OF ACTIVITY—BUT UNDER ADULT CONTROL												
4. SINGLE CHANNEL ATTENTION: UNDER CHILD'S OWN CONTROL												
5. INTEGRATED ATTENTION: FOR SHORT SPELLS												
6. INTEGRATED ATTENTION: WELL CONTROLLED AND SUSTAINED												

CODE: GRADES   COMMENTS:

1. OCCASIONALLY

2. MOST OF THE TIME
   BUT FLUCTUATING

3. STABLE

NAME:

D.O.B.:   DATE:

PERFORMANCE—NON LINGUISTIC														
I VISUAL PERCEPTION														
MATCHING SHAPES														
CIRCLE														
SQUARE														
TRIANGLE														
RECTANGLE														
OVAL														
DIAMOND														
MORE COMPLEX SHAPES														
II CONSTRUCTIONAL TASKS														
1. BUILDING TOWERS														
BUILDING WALLS														
BUILDING BRIDGES														
BUILDING HOUSES														
BUILDING STAIRCASES														
2. COPYING MODELS														
1–4 BRICKS														
4–7 BRICKS														
7 + BRICKS														
3. BLOCK DESIGN														
4–7 BRICKS														
7 + BRICKS														

CODE: GRADES   COMMENTS:

1. OCCASIONALLY

2. MOST OF THE TIME
   BUT FLUCTUATING

3. STABLE

NAME:

D.O.B.:   DATE:

SYMBOLIC UNDERSTANDING												
I OBJECT RECOGNITION												
1. NORMAL SIZE:												
CUP												
SPOON												
BRUSH												
2. SMALL SIZE:												
CUP												
SPOON												
BRUSH												
II LARGE DOLL-PLAY												
1. RECOGNITION BY USE												
2. USE IN IMAGINATIVE PLAY												
III SMALL TOY-PLAY												
1. RECOGNITION BY USE												
2. IMAGINATIVE PLAY												
IV ROLE PLAYING												
V MATCHING (i)												
1. TOY TO PICTURE												
2. PICTURE TO TOY												
VI MATCHING (ii)												
1. GESTURE TO PICTURE												
2. PICTURE TO GESTURE												
VII READING READINESS												

CODE: GRADES
1. OCCASIONALLY
2. MOST OF THE TIME
   BUT FLUCTUATING
3. STABLE

COMMENTS:

NAME:

D.O.B.:   DATE:

CONCEPT FORMATION															
I ONE-TO-ONE MATCHING															
a. COLOURS															
b. SHAPES															
c. OBJECTS															
II CLASSIFICATION															
1. SORTING															
a. COLOURS															
b. SHAPES															
c. OBJECTS															
2. SORTING INTO CATEGORIES BY USE, ETC.															
III SIZE															
1. RELATIVE SIZE OF TWO:															
a. BIG/SMALL															
b. LONG/SHORT															
c. FAT/THIN															
(OR EQUIVALENTS)															
2. SIZE ORDERING OF MORE THAN TWO															
IV QUANTITIES															
1. MORE															
LESS															
SAME															
2. RELATIVE QUANTITIES IN MORE THAN TWO COMPARISONS															

NAME:

D.O.B.:   DATE:

CONCEPT FORMATION													
V POSITIONS													
IN/OUT													
ON													
UP/DOWN													
OVER													
UNDER													
TOP													
NEAR/NEXT TO													
BEHIND													
IN FRONT OF													
BOTTOM													
LEFT/RIGHT													

CODE: GRADES	COMMENTS:
1. OCCASIONALLY	
2. MOST OF THE TIME BUT FLUCTUATING	
3. STABLE	

NAME:

D.O.B.: DATE:

VERBAL COMPREHENSION													
Situational understanding													
VERBAL LABELS													
RELATING 2 NOUNS													
RELATING 2 CONCEPTS: NOUN. VERB													
RELATING 2 CONCEPTS: NOUN. ADJ													
RELATING 3 OR MORE CONCEPTS													

EXPRESSIVE LANGUAGE													
Situational words and phrases													
VERBAL LABELS—NAMING OBJECTS													
RELATING 2 NOUNS													
RELATING 2 CONCEPTS: NOUN. VERB													
RELATING 2 CONCEPTS: NOUN. ADJ													
RELATING 3 OR MORE CONCEPTS													

CODE: GRADES

1. OCCASIONALLY

2. MOST OF THE TIME
   BUT FLUCTUATING

3. STABLE

COMMENTS:

NAME:

D.O.B.:   DATE:

USE OF LANGUAGE:													
COMMUNICATION													
1. ADULT INITIATED a. CHILD RESPONDS NON-VERBALLY													
b. CHILD RESPONDS VERBALLY WHEN COAXED													
c. CHILD RESPONDS READILY TO QUESTIONS, COMMANDS, ETC.													
2. CHILD INITIATED a. ATTENTION SEEKING BY VERBAL MEANS													
b. OFFERS INFORMATION OR COMMENTS													
c. ASKS QUESTIONS, ASKS FOR INFORMATION													
3. CHILD TO CHILD													

CODE: GRADES	COMMENTS:
1. OCCASIONALLY	
2. MOST OF THE TIME BUT FLUCTUATING	
3. STABLE	

NAME:

D.O.B.:   DATE:

USE OF LANGUAGE														
I DIRECTIVE FUNCTION														
1. CANNOT USE DIRECTIVE LANGUAGE														
2. ADULT VERBALIZATION HELPS														
3. CHILD EXTERNALIZES LANGUAGE														
4. LANGUAGE INTERNALIZED														
II IN PLAY														
1. NAMING OBJECTS														
2. VERBAL ACCOMPANIMENT TO PLAY														
3. CHILD EXTERNALIZES LANGUAGE AS INTEGRATIVE FUNCTION														
4. LANGUAGE INTERNALIZED														

CODE: GRADES

1. OCCASIONALLY

2. MOST OF THE TIME BUT FLUCTUATING

3. STABLE

COMMENTS:

References

Conn, P. 1974: The interrelations of alternatives in symbolic representation. *British Journal of Disorders of Communication* 9 (2), 92–100

Cooper, J., Moodley, M. and Reynell, J. 1974: Intervention programmes for pre-school children with delayed language development. *British Journal of Disorders of Communication* 9 (2) 81–91

Crystal, D., Fletcher, P. and Garman, M. 1976: *The Grammatical Analysis of Language Disability. A Procedure in Assessment and Remediation.* London: Edward Arnold

Francis-Williams, J. 1970: *Children with Specific Learning Difficulties.* Oxford: Pergamon Press

Fraser, G. M. and Blockley 1973: The Language Disordered Child. Windsor: NFER Publishing Company

Furth, H. G. 1966: *Thinking without Language.* London: Collier Macmillan Ltd and the Free Press

Griffiths, R. 1970: *The Abilities of Young Children.* London: Child Development Research Centre

Irwin, J. V. and Marge, M. 1972: *Principles of Childhood Language Disabilities.* New York: Appleton-Century-Crofts

Kirk, A. and Kirk, W. D. 1972: *Psycholinguistic Learning Disabilities. Diagnosis and Remediation,* Urbana, Illinois: University of Illinois Press:

Lavatelli, C. S. 1972: *Language Training in Early Childhood Education*: Urbana, Illinois: University of Illinois Press

Lee, L. L., Koenigsknecht, R. A. and Mulhern, S. 1975: *Interactive Language Development Teaching:* Evanston, Illinois: Northern University Press

Lowe, M. 1975: Trends in the development of representational play in infants from one to three years: An observational study. *Journal of Child Psychology and Psychiatry* 16 (1), 33–47

Luria, A. R. 1961: *The Role of Speech in the Regulation of Normal and Abnormal Behaviour* Oxford: Pergamon Press

Piaget, J. 1953: *The Origins of Intelligence in the Child.* London: Routledge and Kegan Paul

Piaget, J. 1974: *The Child's Construction of Quantities.* London: Routledge and Kegan Paul

Von Raffler-Engel, W. and Hutcheson, R. H. 1975: *Language Intervention Programmes in the United States 1960–1974.* Assen/Amsterdam: Van Gorcum & Comp. B.V.

Randall, D., Reynell, J. and Curwen, M. 1974: A study of language development in a sample of 3 year old children. *British Journal of Disorders of Communication* 9 (1) 3–16

Reynell, J. 1969: *Reynell Developmental Language Scales.* Manual. Windsor: NFER Publishing Company

Reynell, J. 1970: Children with physical handicaps. In *The Psychological Assessment of Mental and Physical Handicaps,* ed. Peter Mittler. pp. 459–460, London: Methuen

Reynell, J. 1972: Language handicaps in mentally retarded children. In *Learning, Speech and Thought in the Mentally Retarded,* ed. A. D. B. Clarke and M. M. Lewis. London: Butterworth

Reynell, J. 1976a: Early education for handicapped children. *Child: care, helath and development* **2**, 305–316

Reynell, J. 1976b: Assessment of language development. In *Language and Communication in General Practice,* ed. Bernice Tanner. London: Hodder and Stoughton

Reynell, J. 1977: Unpublished data from the revision of the Reynell Developmental Language Scales.

Ward, D. 1973: A comparative study of children with normal and delayed or deviant language development. Unpublished M.Sc.Thesis, University of London

Index